Psychodynamic Self Psychology in the Treatment of Anorexia and Bulimia

This book presents an implementation of psychodynamic self psychology in the treatment of anorexia nervosa and bulimia nervosa, using a theoretical and therapeutic approach to examine the way that patients turn to food consumption or avoidance to supply needs they do not believe can be provided by human beings.

The book starts with an overview of self psychology, presenting both the theory of self psychology and its specific application for the etiology and treatment of eating disorders. Featuring contributions from eating disorder professionals, the book then integrates this theory with 16 compelling case studies to explore how the eating-disordered patient is scared to take up space in a society that encourages precisely that.

Professionals in the field of psychotherapy for eating disorders, as well as the entire community of psychotherapists, will benefit from the empirical capability of the theory to predict the development as well as remission from eating disorders.

Eytan Bachar, PhD, is Head Psychologist of Hadassah University Medical Center in Jerusalem, Israel; Associate Professor at the Hebrew University of Jerusalem and former chairman of the Israeli Association of Eating Disorders.

Analu Verbin, PhD, is a Clinical Psychologist, working in a private practice in Tel Aviv and a former member of the executive board of the Israeli Association of Eating Disorders.

T0384799

Psychodynamic Self Psychology in the Treatment of Anorexia and Bulimia

Eytan Bachar and Analu Verbin

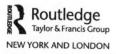

Routledge
Taylor & Francis Group

NEW YORK AND LONDON

First published 2021
by Routledge
52 Vanderbilt Avenue, New York, NY 10017

and by Routledge
2 Park Square, Milton Park, Abingdon, Oxon, OX14 4RN

Routledge is an imprint of the Taylor & Francis Group, an informa business

© 2021 Taylor & Francis

Library of Congress Cataloging-in-Publication Data
Names: Bachar, Eytan, editor. | Verbin, Analu, editor.
Title: Psychodynamic self psychology in the treatment of anorexia and
    bulimia / edited by Eytan Bachar and Analu Verbin.
Description: New York, NY : Routledge, 2021. | Includes
    bibliographical references and index.
Identifiers: LCCN 2020025038 (print) | LCCN 2020025039 (ebook) |
    ISBN 9780367429409 (hardback) | ISBN 9780367336882
    (paperback) | ISBN 9781003000280 (ebook)
Subjects: LCSH: Anorexia nervosa—Treatment. | Bulimia—
    Treatment. | Psychodynamic psychotherapy. | Self psychology.
Classification: LCC RC552.A5 P798 2021 (print) | LCC RC552.A5
    (ebook) | DDC 616.85/262—dc23
LC record available at https://lccn.loc.gov/2020025038
LC ebook record available at https://lccn.loc.gov/2020025039

ISBN: 978-0-367-42940-9 (hbk)
ISBN: 978-0-367-33688-2 (pbk)
ISBN: 978-1-003-00028-0 (ebk)

Typeset in Times
by Apex CoVantage, LLC

Contents

Contributors

Eytan Bachar, PhD Associate professor, Department of Psychology, Hebrew University of Jerusalem; head psychologist, Hadassah University Medical Center, Jerusalem, Israel.

Laura Canetti, PhD Clinical psychologist, supervisor at the Eating Disorders Clinic, Department of Psychiatry, Hadassah University Medical Center, Jerusalem, Israel.

Mira Dana, MA Clinical psychologist, formerly at the Eating Disorders Unit, Rambam Medical Center, Haifa, Israel.

Asher Epstein, PsyD Clinical psychologist, formerly supervisor at the Eating Disorders Unit, Department of Psychiatry, Hadassah University Medical Center, Jerusalem, Israel.

Sara Haramati, MA Clinical psychologist; supervisor at the Eating Disorders Unit, Department of Psychiatry, Hadassah University Medical Center, Jerusalem, Israel.

Michal Man, MA Clinical psychologist, formerly at the Department of Psychiatry, Hadassah University Medical Center, Jerusalem, Israel.

Myrna Milun, MA Clinical psychologist and supervisor, Eating Disorders Unit, Department of Psychiatry, Hadassah University Medical Center, Jerusalem, Israel.

Dina Roth, MD Psychiatrist, formerly at the Child Psychiatry Program, Hadassah University Medical Center, Jerusalem, Israel.

Inbar Sharav-Ifargen, MA Clinical psychologist and supervisor, Eating Disorders Unit, Department of Psychiatry, Hadassah University Medical Center, Jerusalem, Israel.

Varda Shavit Ohayon, MA Clinical psychologist, formerly at the Department of Psychiatry, Hadassah University Medical Center, Jerusalem, Israel.

Yael Steinberg, MA Clinical psychologist, formerly at the Department of Psychiatry, Hadassah University Medical Center, Jerusalem, Israel.

Analu Verbin, PhD Clinical psychologist, private clinic, Tel Aviv. Formerly at the Eating Disorders Unit, Department of Psychiatry, Hadassah University Medical Center, Jerusalem, Israel.

Preface

In recent decades, anorexia and bulimia have become one of the most frightening nightmares, mainly of affluent societies, particularly within the risk population: adolescent girls and early adult women. Young females suffering from these disorders bring themselves to the verge of death or to radical restriction of existence both in the physical and psychological sense. This is particularly striking in a society that opens up for these young women opportunities for growth, self-expression and occupying meaningful space in the world.

This book presents the theory of self psychology, the insights it offers as to the origins and etiology of eating disorders and therapeutic techniques. The first part presents the theory, its empirical examination and its application to eating disorders. The second part presents 16 case studies in 15 chapters. Each chapter describes in detail a specific treatment, typically from the beginning to the conclusion, while integrating the principles derived from self psychology and their application in therapy.

The first part consists of four chapters. The first chapter presents the history of diagnosis and treatment of eating disorders. This chapter also covers issues of epidemiology and prevention, both in their general medical context and from the specific perspective of self psychology. Finally, it compares self psychology to other contemporary approaches while highlighting parallel insights.

The second chapter discusses the fundamentals of self psychology and the application of these principles in the treatment of anorexia and bulimia. It presents over 20 clinical vignettes that illustrate the opportunities and dilemmas arising from the application of self psychology in the treatment of eating disorders.

The third chapter presents the evidence basis for the application of psychodynamic self psychology in eating disorders.

The fourth chapter then concludes the theory and research part of the book. It describes the complexity of managing the treatment in the entanglement of transference, countertransference, real risks posed by the patient's physical condition and interactions with other team members from various disciplines.

The second part consists of 15 chapters, each presenting a clinical case study. The clinical cases were contributed by professionals supervised by the first author of the present book, Eytan Bachar, both clinically and theoretically. The contributed cases were evaluated and refined by him to create the scientific unity of the book. All of the treatments were conducted in Israel, which is representative in rates and distribution of eating disorders to the US and other Western countries. The total majority of the cases were conducted at Hadassah University Medical Center in Jerusalem, and one at the Rambam Medical Center in Haifa. All identifying details of the patients were concealed to protect their privacy.

Ten of these chapters present anorexic patients and five present bulimic patients. In all cases, improvement was achieved throughout the therapy, ranging from small improvements to full remission. This matches our evaluation that once the patient manages to "harness" herself to therapy, to create a working alliance with the therapist and persist in therapy, positive change is most likely to occur. This is also consistent with the empirical evidence presented in Chapter 3. However, we also bear in mind those patients who dropped from therapy after one or two sessions, before meaningful relationship and alliance could be constituted. They are not represented in this book, as they have never allowed us to get to know them. The dropout rate in our clinics is similar to the rates reported in the world, between 20 and 25 percent of the referrals.

Significant parts of the present book were previously published by the first author in Hebrew in Israel. Analu Verbin, the second author of the present book, translated these parts to English and participated in updating and editing the book.

During the last 20 years, research has provided ample support for the insights of psychodynamic self psychology and its effectiveness in the treatment of eating disorders. This research proves the capability of the theory of psychodynamic self psychology to predict in cross-sectional and prospective longitudinal studies, both the development of and the remission from eating disorders. In addition, it showed the effectiveness of psychodynamic self psychological treatment in a randomized control study over two other techniques.

Returning to some of the cases that were published in the Hebrew version, as well as presenting three out of the four new case studies that were added here, enabled us to observe long-term achievements and persistence of recovery, even up to ten years.

We would like to thank our colleagues who have shared their experience and contributed case studies. Special thanks go to Linor Levi for her invaluable logistic and research assistance, and to Sara Gladstone and Adina Wolff Ciner for their linguistic contributions. We would also like to thank Myrna Milun, who gave us additional linguistic support, in addition to the two case studies that she contributed. We also thank Jonathan Nadav, head of Magnes Press, for his support. Finally, we thank Amanda Devine and Grace McDonnell from Routledge for their instrumental and kind help in seeing the book to publication.

Eytan Bachar   Analu Verbin

Part I

Theory, Application and Empirical Evidence

1   Anorexia and Bulimia

Diagnosis and History of Treatment

Eytan Bachar

Anorexia nervosa (AN) is one of the most severe, and at the same time most peculiar and intriguing, mental illnesses. With no other mental or cognitive disorder other than body perception distortions, a perfectly capable and intelligent young woman, often particularly bright, starves herself, sometimes to death. Bulimia nervosa (BN) was distinctively defined as a separate diagnosis only in the early 1980s (American Psychiatric Association, 1980). Anorexia and bulimia are sister-disorders, with a spectrum of disorders in between, whose symptoms are a mixture of those two clinical pictures. Whereas a girl diagnosed with restrictive AN maintains her low body weight by restricting her food intake, a girl diagnosed with BN maintains such weight through active purging of the food after having consumed massive amounts of it. Purging food after bingeing is typically through vomiting or excessive physical activity. An alternative purging method is through laxatives; although this method does not in fact contribute to losing weight since it accelerates purging after the food is already digested. Fifty percent of the patients diagnosed with BN have been anorexic in the past. In this book, we will refer to patients in the female form, since women and girls make up around 90 percent of those diagnosed with AN or BN.

Diagnosis

The DSM cites in its fifth edition (APA, 2013) the list of symptoms and indications necessary for diagnosing AN or BN.

Diagnostic Criteria of Anorexia Nervosa

1.   Restriction of energy intake relative to requirements leading to a significantly low body weight in the context of age, sex, developmental trajectory and physical health. Significantly low weight is

defined as a weight that is less than minimally normal or, for children and adolescents, less than minimally expected.
2. Intense fear of gaining weight or becoming fat, or persistent behavior that interferes with weight gain, even though at a significantly low weight.
3. Disturbance in the way in which one's body weight or shape is experienced, undue influence of body weight or shape on self-evaluation or persistent lack of recognition of the seriousness of the current low body weight.

Specific Subtypes of Anorexia

Restrictive Type – when for over three months, the patient has not experienced binge eating episodes or purging behavior (by vomits, abuse of laxatives, diuretics or enemas).
Bingeing/Purging Type – when for over three months, the patient has experienced recurrent episodes of bingeing or purging.

Diagnostic Criteria of Bulimia Nervosa

1. Recurrent episodes of binge eating. An episode of binge eating is characterized by *both* of the following:

   A. Eating in a discrete amount of time (e.g., within a two-hour period) an amount of food that is definitely larger than what most individuals would eat in a similar period of time under similar circumstances.
   B. Sense of lack of control over eating during an episode.

2. Recurrent inappropriate compensatory behavior to prevent weight gain, such as self-induced vomiting; misuse of laxatives, diuretics or other medications; fasting; or excessive exercise.
3. The binge eating and inappropriate compensatory behaviors both occur, on average, at least once a week for three months.
4. Self-evaluation is unduly influenced by body shape and weight.
5. The disturbance does not occur exclusively during episodes of anorexia nervosa.

Physical Complications of AN and BN

An anorexic patient's bodily complications are a result of the extreme starvation and the subsequent thinness. One major complication that even comprised one of the diagnostic criteria in the past is *amenorrhea*

– that is the cessation of menstruation in menstruating women. Additional complications are constipation, severe abdominal pains, slowness, low body temperature and failure to thrive to the body's full potential. Some patients develop "lanugo," thin hair on their hands and buttocks. This is the body's attempt to maintain its temperature, which is decreasing due to lack of minimum layers of fat. Other physical symptoms are skin dryness, cold intolerance and low pulse. If normal eating restoration is not gradual, severe edema may appear. Bone density may also significantly decrease. Death rate of AN is estimated at over 10 percent. Most physical complications of BN stem from the self-inflicted vomiting, including severe damage to the teeth, esophagus, saliva glands and balance of fluids and electrolytes, sometimes causing potentially fatal heart complications. However, death rate of BN is unknown. Amenorrhea is rarer in BN than in AN because body weight in BN stays closer to normal, with slight deviations. The reason for amenorrhea in BN is not entirely clear yet.

Distribution

The rate of anorexia in the risk population is 0.5 percent–1 percent of all late adolescent girls and young adult women. The rate of bulimia in the same population is 1 percent to 3 percent.

Both anorexia and bulimia are much more prevalent in rich and industrialized societies with an abundance of food. Developing world immigrants to rich countries may develop the disorder in rates similar to local populations. Furthermore, in rich countries the disorder is more common in higher socioeconomic levels than in lower socioeconomic groups (Hsu, 1990). Research of the difference in distribution across socioeconomic levels was published in the Netherlands in 1998 (Hoek, 1998), indicating that the rate of bulimia is seven times higher in the Netherlands' urban areas than in its rural areas. Hsu (1990) reports an interesting finding regarding the Arab Emirates: the rate of eating disorders in those emirates was increasing in direct relationship to improvement in quality of life and income level, up to seven times higher. His observations show a kind of social contagion within high school classes or cohorts where a case of anorexia was found – one case leads to additional cases. All those findings indicate the crucial influence of social, cultural and psychological factors on the rates of eating disorders. At the same time, certain genetic risk factors might increase the chances of an eating disorder to emerge. It is known that in families of anorexic or bulimic patients, the frequency of nutrition problems (ranging from obesity to anorexia), or of other mental illnesses is higher (APA,

1994). The genetic factor's impact on the disorder's course is yet to be explored, or its contribution, if at all, to the statistically explained variance of these disorders.

Traditionally, the common age for the onset of anorexia or bulimia had been adolescence or early adulthood, with the average onset age being 17. It was very rare to find such disorders before adolescence, or after 40, and some even suggested a bipolar curve of onset in age 14 or 18. However, in recent years it appears that the age range is expanding, as more prepubescent girls are being admitted to both inpatients and outpatient facilities, even at the age of nine or ten. The average onset age for bulimia is slightly older (more inclined toward late adolescence and early young adulthood). This phenomenon is also in line with the fact that at least in 50 percent of bulimia cases, the disorder emerged after the patient has already suffered from anorexia.

The duration of the disease is varied in both disorders. Some patients recover after a short period of time (several months), and some are drawn into the disease for years. Strober (1998) published a prolonged observation of anorexic patients over more than 15 years. He found that after six years of treatment, 65 percent of the patients were fully recovered and none of them relapsed back to the disease; another 12 percent were in partial recovery, and 10 percent of them relapsed; 13 percent were not recovered even after six years of treatment.

History of the Treatment of Anorexia

As early as the late seventeenth century, the medical literature saw a report of a disease matching the description of anorexia (Morton, 1694). Until the early 1930s, at least seven articles were published proposing that anorexia has physical origins and suggesting mineral salts and different kinds of baths as a cure. While Sigmund Freud pointed out the psychic origins of anorexia already in 1895 (Breuer & Freud, 1895; Freud, Bonaparte, Freud, & Kris, 1954), it wasn't until the 1930s that the psychological origin of the disorder was acknowledged, and psychotherapy increasingly became the central route for treatment.

Psychoanalysis, undoubtedly the leading theory in the field of psychotherapy, has developed from the beginning of the twentieth century and to this day has three distinct models to understand pathology and normality of the human psyche. Like in any other science, each new psychoanalytic model encompasses its predecessors. Scholars and therapists treating anorexia (bulimia was defined as a distinctive syndrome only since the 1980s) were using the "lenses" and the "map" provided by the dominant model of the time. Thus, since the 1930s to early 1950s, scholars and professionals treating anorexia observed the disorder through the prism of the drive-defense model. According to this model, underlying the psychic life is a conflict between sexual and aggressive drives and a strict "super ego." The "ego" exercises defense mechanisms to mediate between them. This model is effective in neurotic patients since their psychic structures are in order. However, anorexic patients do not appear to be driven by strong impulses. Sexuality seems to be the last thing on their mind. On the contrary, they seem to have annihilated drives. But since the therapists of the time had only the lenses and concepts of the drive-defense model, these concepts were applied to anorexia. Moulton (1942) and Waller, Kaufman, and Deutsch (1940) proposed that self-starvation is a defense from fantasies of oral impregnation. Masserman (1941) suggested that the pervasive refusal to eat is a defense from sadistic-cannibalistic oral fantasies. This model did not make a significant contribution to the treatment of anorexia both because of its theoretical presumptions and its interpretative and confrontative technique that was ill-fitted to treating these girls.

The drive-defense model contends that the tension between the sexual and aggressive drives on the one hand, and the strict super ego on the other hand, generates the neurotic symptoms. But the model fails to account for a major part of the anorexic and bulimic symptoms. The distorted body perception, the alienation from internal feelings and the paralyzing fear of self-realization indicate a more severe damage to the psychic structure than a conflict between structured psychic systems. As mentioned earlier, in many cases anorexic and bulimic patients exhibit avoidance of sexuality. But it ensues not out of fear or guilt because of the Oedipal complex, but the fear of growing up. Growing up means abandoning the girl's position of special attunement to her parents, which we'll later explore in detail. In the sixth chapter, we'll see the case of an anorexic girl who was disappointed and discouraged by her father's reaction to her growing up. She felt he was hoping for her to stay slim, small and angel-like and that her signs of sexual development made him sad because he did not want them to grow apart. He used a Hebrew expression that literally makes a comment about the size of her bottom, which both points out the sexual markers and disapproves of her exhibiting her presence, both physically and behaviorally. Whereas the neurotic patient feels guilty about the pleasure she derives from satisfying wishes she deems forbidden, the anorexic or bulimic patient feels guilty about feeling any form of pleasure. This is because of her inability to attend to herself, to care for herself and satisfy her own needs, characteristics which we'll further elaborate in the next chapters. In the advanced phases of the treatment, after a stronger self is built, the patient may exhibit sexual preoccupations with Oedipal tones. At this point, the treatment would resemble a classic treatment of neurosis. Such early signs of Oedipal elements in the advanced phases of treatment can be found in Chapters 16 and 17.

The object-relations model is the next layer in the development of psychoanalysis. This model is concerned with the modes of attachment between individuals. It contains the first model since a large part of such human attachment is about sexual and aggressive drives. But apart from the psychosexual developmental axis, Mahler (1968) has outlined an additional developmental axis based on her observations. The steps along this axis were not the stages of the psychosexual development, but stages of the psychological development allowing a child to gradually separate herself from her mother. Scholars and practitioners who used the object-relations model to treat anorexia – Masterson (1995); Sours (1980); Selvini-Palazzoli (1985) – described the strains of separation of the anorexic patients. The difficulties of separation according to this model are reflected in the anorexic patient in severe disgust of her mother's figure. To avoid resembling her mother, for instance in her femininity, the anorexic girl mutilates her own body. By that she symbolically annihilates the internalized mother figure. The treatment technique in this model, like its preceding model, is interpretation that often acquires a confrontational tone. Interpretations and confrontations are adequate for treating an unsolved conflict better than for filling in and repairing deficiencies in the self. Goodsitt (1997), a self psychology scholar and practitioner, points out that neither in the case studies of the previously cited scholars nor in his own cases could he find evidence for confusion of the anorexic patient's self-perception and the figure of her mother; and particularly not that such confusion is intermediated by oral fantasies.

The difficulty of the anorexic or bulimic patient to separate is only a part of the broader explanation provided by self psychology. Self psychology discusses not only the difficulty of separation, but also the difficulty of individuation, namely, reluctance to develop an independent individuum that is an independent center of initiative and promote its own interests.

Self psychology is the third layer of psychoanalysis. Kohut (1971) described an additional developmental axis: the narcissistic axis. Along this axis, narcissistically relying on others is not one single developmental stage from which the mature individual grows up and totally abandons this stage like in the object-relations axis. Kohut's theory legitimizes this human need all through one's life. The healthy development along this axis is moving from a total and desperate reliance on others to a flexible and mature reliance.

An optimal fostering environment allows the baby or the toddler an appropriate narcissistic reliance. This is reliance where the person on whom one relies is willing to give up his or her needs and viewpoint and act from the relying person's perspective. By this he or she acts as a selfobject, a term we'll discuss in detail in the next chapter. In such conditions, the child develops a strong and healthy self who is capable of exercising from within the soothing and regulation mechanism previously exercised from without, by the selfobject. This process advances while fluctuating between empathic-enough environment to optimal empathic failures. A girl developing an eating disorder does not believe she can rely on other people to fulfill her selfobject needs. Throughout her growing up years, a role reversal is taking place between parent and child: the parent is the one to narcissistically rely on the child rather than the other way around. When the parent thus relies on the child, namely, expects the child to attend to the parent and fulfills the parent's needs (for example, needs of soothing, consolation and regulation of depressive feelings), rather than to act as having interests and perspective of her own, the child might feel as if she has no right to live her own life, and in this sense she is selfless, lacking a self. Such children, who devote themselves to the prosperity of their parents while negating their own internal needs and who do not believe that another person can fulfill their selfobject needs, tend to develop eating disorders (Goodsitt, 1985, 1997). When a girl feels selfless, she experiences self-guilt whenever she attempts to act for her own sake, since her role, as she perceives it, is to attend to her parents and fulfill their needs. Later on, in the transference process well-known in psychology, she would feel obliged to fulfill the needs of other significant people in her life. The reason for this is that independent thinking and feeling are experienced as betrayal of the person whose selfobject needs she must fulfill. She feels self-guilt about occupying a psychological space in the world, namely, self-expression, presence, will and opinion. She experiences all these as immoral, destructive and harmful to others. This self-guilt also accounts for her will not to occupy a physical space in the world, therefore not to eat. Eating means providing for the self and attending to internal sources of need, as opposed to attending to external duties (Goodsitt, 1985). Eating also reflects acknowledgment of her right to consider her own interests and prioritize herself over others. Eating thus becomes a selfish act for the anorexic or bulimic girl. The bulimic patient will purge what she ate because she experiences the binge as an indecent act of self-indulgence. The anorexic patient perceives eating itself as an unjustified act that expresses self-indulgence, betraying the role of serving as a selfobject for others.

These central characteristics of the eating-disordered patient, namely, self-guilt and self-deprecation, also generate what psychoanalytic literature terms "negative therapeutic reaction." Recovery would lead to self-advancement and a sense of psychic presence, which as mentioned earlier she perceives as betrayal and as inappropriate stance.

The picture depicted of the anorexic or bulimic girl is a picture of a deficit in the sense of self. Only self psychology, which conceptualizes such deficit of the self, can explain feelings of lack of self-initiative, self-alienation, lack of enthusiasm and lack of vitality.

The self psychologically oriented therapist exercises a special therapeutic stance that emphasizes attunement to the needs of the self. In the next chapter, we'll elaborate how the self psychology therapist revives in this manner the patient's depleted and undeveloped self. Through this therapeutic stance, the therapist renews or activates the patient's belief that she can rely on another person to fulfill her selfobject needs, instead of on substance (food, either by consuming it or avoiding it).

In Chapter 3, we will present several empirical papers providing the evidence base for self psychology in eating disorders. We will present papers showing positive correlation between the extent of selflessness and the severity of the eating disorder symptoms. Also, we will present studies showing the capability of the theory of psychodynamic self psychology to predict in cross-sectional and prospective longitudinal studies, both the development of and the remission from eating disorders. In addition, we will present the effectiveness of psychodynamic self psychological treatment in a randomized control study over two other techniques.

Self Psychology Compared to Other Contemporary Approaches

Self psychology conceptualization of anorexia and bulimia is close to clinical observations and conceptualizations of other psychological approaches. The therapeutic techniques, observation tools and the therapist's stance vary across approaches, but it is fascinating to trace down the similar perception of etiology, observations and conceptualization across such different and often opposite approaches. Such resemblance further validates the perception of the underlying problem.

Within psychoanalysis, the Kleinian approach is considered opposite to self psychology. Nevertheless, neo-Kleinian theorists such as Williams have conceptualized eating disorders in a way that strikingly resembles the conceptualization of self psychology. Williams (1997) describes a reversal of roles of container and contained between the future eating-disordered girl and her parents. According to this approach, the mother cannot exercise for her child what Bion (1959) calls alpha functioning, which is the parent's capacity to contain the daughter's harsh emotions and mitigate them. The mother of the future eating-disordered girl, Williams contends, cannot fulfill such functions for her child, and moreover, she projects her own harsh feelings onto the child and expects the latter to contain them. Validation for such an argument may be found in self psychology's observations and concept of reversed self-selfobject roles between parents and children. The range of selfobject's functions and roles is much broader than mere containment functions, the focus of Bion and Williams, but containment is surely a major part thereof.

Andre Green (2001), who does not use the theoretical tools of self psychology, provides further support for the self psychological approach by proposing that the AN patient is characterized by what he terms "negative narcissism" or "death narcissism" by reducing her being. A similar view can be found in Lacanian school, for example, Fink (2016).

On the other "pole" of psychoanalysis, relational psychoanalysts highlight the role of trauma and dissociation in the etiology of eating disorders, generally suggesting that the eating disorder symptoms hold dissociated parts of the patient's self (Bromberg, 2006; Petrucelli, 2015). Yet within this framework, relational psychoanalysts adopt self psychology's conceptualization of food as selfobject and acknowledge that it provides the eating-disordered patient with the selfobject function of soothing and comfort, allowing self-regulation (Petrucelli, 2015).

The cognitive behavioral therapy (CBT) approach in psychology is considered opposite to all psychoanalytic strands. However, it is fascinating to see once again that when it comes to underlying characteristics of eating disorders and the respective therapeutic objectives, CBT goes hand in hand with the modern version of psychoanalysis embodied in self psychology. Garner and Garfinkel (1985) consider low self-esteem, inability to stand for one's opinion and inability to express one's wishes features that may predict anorexia. In cognitive behavioral treatment of anorexia (which is largely untreated by CBT compared to bulimia, in which cognitive behavioral treatment is much more frequent), Garner and Garfinkel suggest rewarding the anorexic girl anytime she demonstrates behaviors expressing her own will.

Family therapy (Minuchin, Rosman, & Baker, 1978; Selvini-Palazzoli, 1985) also attempts, however differently than self psychology or CBT, to release the girl of the enmeshment and overprotectiveness of her family. Through improving family communication, family therapy would attempt to allow the anorexic girl to search for her autonomous will and articulate it. Family therapists, for instance (Selvini-Palazzoli, 1985), may instruct the entire family to listen for ten minutes to the girl, who in turn was instructed to state only what she autonomously wants and chooses rather than what she wants for other family members.

Finally, conceptual similarities to the self psychological ideas can be found in research borrowing from other concepts. Using narrative research, Wechselblatt and colleagues concluded that women encouraged by their families to substitute others' needs for their own are at elevated risk for developing AN (Wechselblatt, Gurnick, & Simon, 2000). Certain personality traits like compliance and perfectionism render them especially susceptible to their family's pressure to attune to the needs of others. The future anorexic subsequently negates her right to need and to be nourished.

The concept of survival guilt was expanded by Modell (1971), in terms that support the fundamental understandings of self psychology. Modell described the belief of an anorexic patient that the supply of good things in life is limited and that drawing on it deprives others, primarily close relatives, causing them to suffer. If eating-disordered patients believe that success and happiness are achieved at the expense of others, they will tend to give up their portion. We present a similar vignette in Chapter 15.

In the research field of narcissism, Brunton, Lacey and Waller (2005) found an association in a nonclinical population between drive for thinness and a construct remarkably similar to selflessness, "narcissistically abused personality," defined as the placing of others' needs before one's own.

Why Women?

The vast majority of anorexia and bulimia patients, around 90 percent, are women. The fact that 10 percent of the patients are men shows that the disorder cannot be accounted for only by body shape or female hormones. The occurrence of both anorexia and bulimia in men also questions the ability of earlier models – drive-defense and object-relations models – to account for these disorders, since it is not expected that men would beware of oral impregnation or fear resembling the mother's body.

What, then, are the psychological and sociological explanation for this striking majority of women within eating-disordered patients? The simple explanation, pointing to how the Western fashion industry encourages women to be slim, cannot fully account for the disorder. First, reports of anorexia are evident for over three centuries, including the early 1900s when the female beauty ideal was not yet dominated by thinness. Second, in the same society with the same fashion influence, only 1 percent and 3 percent of the girls in the risk age group develop anorexia and bulimia, respectively. Furthermore, there are other societies, such as the Chinese, whose ideal of female beauty is also thin, but in which anorexia and bulimia are scarce. Contrary to Western prevalent belief, scholars have reported that classic and contemporary Chinese literature as well as past and present public opinion are all inclined to favor the slim female ideal (Leung, David, & Cheung, 1998). And yet, anorexia and bulimia are not as prevalent in China as they are in Western societies, probably because China is not an affluent society. One must have an abundance of food to be able to "play" with it to communicate symbolic and mental articulations. "Affluence" does not refer to the material abundance of food alone; however, it is clearly important to be able to use it symbolically either by avoiding it or by consuming and purging it.

"Affluence" also means affluence of opportunities for self-expression and self-advancement. Levin (1994); Levin and Smolak (1992); and Silverstein and Perlick (1995) comment that eating disorders are more frequent in societies that, on the one hand, open up opportunities for women to develop and express themselves, and, on the other hand, still expect women to serve others, primarily their husbands or other family members. The Western society, along with its affluence of food, not only allows but praises individualism and self-cultivation. The anorexic girl experiences her choice of individualism as a sin, or as something she is not worthy of. In this regard, Tchanturia and Katzman (2000) found that once the country of Georgia opened up to the multiple opportunities and choices of a capitalist society, the rate of eating disorders increased. Along the same veins, Gluck (2000), who studied the Jewish community in the US, found that secular women were twice as dissatisfied by their body shape and inclined to eating disorders as ultra-orthodox women. One can argue that it may be that women's gender role in the ultra-orthodox society is clearer and more defined, and she is less familiar with the opportunity to take up space, with freedom of choice or with individualism.

Adolescence is a risk period for the anorexia-prone girl: bodily signals emerge and indicate the end of childhood and the beginning of adulthood, a chapter that generates and calls for taking up space and asserting presence, tasks that she feels do not befit her. It is not sexuality, separation or femininity per se that frighten the anorexic girl, as earlier theoreticians suggested, but something much more holistic: a full life in the affluent society. Men in the same society are not encouraged to deprecate themselves and are not rewarded, whether explicitly or implicitly, for giving up their space. On the contrary, boys and men are rewarded for behaviors of self-advancement and breaking through, and even for aggressively pushing others aside. Kearney-Cooke (1991) found in her study that men who do not act in correspondence with the expected stereotype, namely, men who do not stand up for their opinions, passively give in to others' will and do not express their wishes, manifest higher rate of eating disorders compared to the general male population. In the next part of the book, we'll describe a case of an adolescent boy giving up himself and his needs in the service of his parents' needs, mainly his mother's, and this led to his eating disorder.

A simple but interesting research on students' associations as to the size of a lady's meal may be supportive of such conclusions. Chaiken and Pliner (1987) found that students of both sexes perceived a small-sized meal as feminine, and she who eats a small meal was perceived as more polite and considerate. A woman who eats large meals, however, was perceived as unattractive, less polite and less considerate of others. Meals for males were completely free of such associated values. This striking finding demonstrates how both sexes expect women to show less self-presence and to give in satisfying her own needs, and how both sexes associate this kind of behavior to consideration and politeness. Furthermore, expression of such expectations, in both sexes, was directly linked to restricting food intake of women.

It is possible that for women, if they need or seek substances to satisfy self needs, food would be an appropriate choice to meet expectations for more reserved and introvert behavior because handling food is typically more private and easily concealed than using substances such as alcohol or drugs.

It may also be the case that this specific use of the body as a vehicle to manage psychic pain is more characteristic of women than men. In self psychology terms, Sands (2003) suggests that men and women employ different strategies to manage the psychic pain that develops when basic needs are chronically frustrated and that an eating disorder is a "particularly female" solution to disavow the unmet narcissistic needs through literally disavowing bodily needs. In other words, not only that girls are less encouraged than boys to exert their selfhood, or that such encouragement is conflictual at best, as explained earlier, they are more likely than boys to concretize their unmet needs in their own body through disordered eating.

The female dominance made eating disorders an intriguing phenomenon for feminist scholars as well. While early feminist critique highlighted the connection between eating disorders and the cultural ideal of thinness (Boskind-Lodahl, 1976), feminist writers of the 1990s rejected this somewhat one-dimensional understanding of eating disorders and increasingly pointed out the contradictory message they convey. Indeed, since the 1990s, feminist scholars from both social sciences and humanities have shared a common understanding of eating disorders as a demonstration of conflicting values and confusing gender norms (Orbach, 1986; Macsween, 1993; Bordo, 1993). This understanding goes hand in hand with the self psychology approach that locates the origin of eating disorders in a deficit of the self against a backdrop of individualism and affluence of opportunities, as described previously. Feminist psychotherapist Susie Orbach (1986) suggests that one of the major therapeutic goals is "restarting the development of a self," interestingly capturing the essence of self psychology treatment of eating disorders.

Psychotherapy Combined With Metabolic/Nutritional Treatment

As early as the late 1960s and early 1970s, Hilde Bruch (1973) suggested combining psychological treatment with metabolic/nutritional counseling. Goodsitt (1985), one of the pioneering self psychology scholars in the field of anorexia and bulimia, also highlighted the importance of such a combination.

Nutritional/metabolic counseling has three goals. The first is to observe and monitor the patient's physical condition in order to recognize risks that may reach fatal complications or irreversible damage. The psychologist or the nutritionist must see that the patient meets with a metabolic physician who is an eating disorders specialist. This physician will monitor biochemistry and other labs, especially those that pertain to electrolytes, proteins, bone density and body mass index, all parameters that may dictate hospitalization, sometimes emergency hospitalization. Supplementing the diet with the deficient minerals and vitamins are crucial elements for the treatment.

The second goal is to gradually increase the caloric intake for anorexic patients and find a nutritional composition that would support reduction of binges for bulimic patients.

The third goal is to provide patients with healthy eating habits, namely, regular and diverse meals throughout the day. It is important for the nutritionist to provide such habits gradually, that is, increasing the number and content of meals for anorexic patients, and reducing the binges and vomiting for bulimic patients. It is advisable that the psychologist encourage the patient to attend the nutritional/metabolic counseling. In case of total rejection of such counseling, the psychological treatment should be halted or even not started to begin with.

Apart from the necessary contribution of nutritional counseling to overall physical health, it also helps the psychotherapist by releasing him or her from dedicating therapeutic resources to direct monitoring of the bodily symptom. However, there are many cases in which the therapist himself or herself needs to explain to the patient her medical condition and provide guidance regarding healthy eating habits. Such intervention is particularly possible at the beginning of treatment, when the patient's physical condition is still severe and her need to feel "held" is great. The patient's sense of "holding" is also greater because she has additional staff members taking care of her. In these early phases of treatment, many patients require massive time to harness themselves to the therapeutic process. As elaborated in the next chapter, this is because the patients rely on substance (the food) to satisfy their selfobject needs and thus their attachment to the therapist to fulfill these needs is slow. Some are also characterized by what we may title "alexithymia," the inability to express emotions. The therapist's willingness to be more active during these phases and use parameters like encouragement and reassurance that are typically outside the psychodynamic arsenal may contribute to the treatment at this point. In addition, the ability to focus and highlight certain core points in the therapeutic process, which are provided by self psychology (and which will be elaborated upon in the next chapter), may well enhance the patient's feeling that she is "held" and understood.

Many patients refuse to attend treatment at these early stages. The existence of several staff members – psychologist, nutritionist and a metabolic doctor – makes for additional degrees of freedom in choosing the therapeutic point of venture that would later be complemented by the other realms, but only as long as the patients know in advance and agree in principle that the additional dimensions of treatment would be added soon enough. The symptom thus allows them to demonstrate, however distortedly, their autonomy and rebelliousness. This autonomy is obviously very sad since without external holding, it may end up in death.

Prevention

Prevention of a psychological disorder is far more complicated and challenging than prevention of physical illnesses. Whereas the latter may do with a single injection of an immunization, a psychological disorder requires a prolonged and intricate process of preparation and education. Moreover, since a bodily injection is easy to administer, it is quite simple to immunize a large population for research purposes and then observe minor percentage fluctuations (which may be the entire rate of the disease in question) in a broad population. A "psychological immunization" is far more complex and difficult to administer in large populations. This is the reason that our current knowledge of preliminary prevention of anorexia and bulimia is scarce. "Preliminary prevention" means reducing the number of new cases joining the sick population. A meta-analysis (Fingeret, Warren, Cepeda-Benito, & Gleaves, 2006) found that eating disorder prevention programs yielded mixed results, and they are somewhat controversial. Overall, prevention programs have a large effect on improving knowledge and a small effect on reducing maladaptive eating attitudes and behaviors (Fingeret et al., 2006). However, Israeli researchers (Neumark, Butler, & Palti, 1995) found in such prevention study that nutritional education teaching healthy nutrition habits reduced vomiting or risky diets in the trial group compared to control group who did not receive such education.

Any prevention plan consists of two elements: decreasing risk factors and increasing resistance factors. A severe diet in adolescents is undoubtedly a significant risk factor (Hsu, 1990). Parents must therefore be attuned and prevent severe diets while encouraging healthy eating habits of regular and diverse meals. Mass media may doubly contribute to this cause: first by encouraging additional routes for female success other than physical appearance (Levin & Smolak, 1992; Levin, 1994); and second by discouraging loss of weight. Promoting an "ideal of thinness" in mass media renders the early and crucial diagnosis of anorexia much harder.

Cultivating resistance factors is even more challenging. Levin (1994) suggests the promotion of factors generally known as mental immunizations, including self-esteem and self-identity. Self psychology may provide parents with guidance as to more specific resistance factors. According to self psychology, parents must be aware of a girl deprecating herself, her needs, selfhood and acts to meet the needs of others. They should discourage her from doing so, even if such behavior is convenient for them. The best way to accomplish such a goal is to guarantee that parents avoid relying on their daughters to satisfy their own needs of self-esteem, reassurance and regulation of painful emotions. Furthermore, parents should pay attention to their daughter's ability to lean on others. Can she turn to others when she experiences distress or pain? Can she turn to them in times of need and ask for help and support?

Beside that awareness that is required on the parents' part of any possible signs of illness in their daughters, it is equally important to know when this is not the case. Not any thin girl is anorexic. Diagnostic criteria indicate that for an anorexia diagnosis to be given, thinness must be the result of the girl's refusal to gain weight. She must display tremendous anxiety about gaining weight and be considerably preoccupied with this anxiety and with caloric calculations. She must also suffer from distorted body perception, namely, to terribly complain about how fat she is when in fact she is extremely thin. Furthermore, for the diagnosis to be given she must indicate that her self-esteem is influenced by her weight. If these criteria are not met and it is simply thinness of a girl who normally eats regular and diverse meals, there is probably nothing to worry about. In this case, parents should only maintain the healthy eating habits (regular meals with various kinds of food) and gently try to advance, even without words, weight gain – for instance by recognizing the foods she would like. If the low weight is consistent despite the absence of criteria and arrests her development over time, then it is recommended to approach psychological-nutritional counseling.

While thinness is not necessarily a clear-cut sign of anorexia, an initiated and planned vomiting for purging a meal is always a significant and unequivocal sign for an eating disorder. This last remark is particularly important since many patients, especially in the early stages of the disorder, do not fully understand the severity of this behavior. Throwing up seems to them like an effective and harmless "trick" to get rid of calories. They do not understand that this purging action is one of the symptoms of a severe mental illness. Vomiting is such a crucial element of bulimia for a reason; it facilitates the generation of the sick addiction cycle. The patient believes that this "instrument" she has at her disposal allows her to eat even more, and that increases her binge eating. It is also worth mentioning that vomiting never purges *all* calories that were taken in. Moreover, sometimes patients "must" eat more to be able to throw up, which once again facilitates the disordered vicious circle. When parents or other caretakers of the girl suspect an eating disorder, they should hurry and bring her to treatment. The earlier the treatment is, both in anorexia and bulimia, the better the chances to heal.

2 The Emergence of Self Psychology

Opportunities and Dilemmas in the Treatment of Anorexia and Bulimia

Eytan Bachar

The theoretical conceptualizations of self psychology and the ensuing implications for the therapeutic stance open up new opportunities for the treatment of anorexia and bulimia. This chapter presents these opportunities as well as the dilemmas stemming from implementing self psychology, illustrated through clinical vignettes (Bachar, 1998).

The fragility of the anorexic or bulimic patient and her tendency to dismiss her needs, feelings and interests mandate the application of a psychotherapeutic approach that would not impose an interpretation "from without," but rather provide an experience-near "from within" attunement to the patient. Self psychologically informed therapists, more often traditional or classic psychoanalytically oriented therapists, deviate from the free-floating attention technique prescribed by psychoanalysis in favor of special attention and attunement for vicarious introspection into a patient's sense of self. Special attention is given to the patient's experience of the therapist's impact on the patient's sense of self.

According to Wolf (1988), the patient in self psychologically oriented psychotherapy feels the therapist maintains an attuned stance rather than an adversarial one. The patient thus experiences the therapist's neutrality as benign; that is, the therapist is affectively on the side of the patient's self, without necessarily adhering to all of the patient's judgments and assessments. The therapist, according to Kohut (1984) experiences herself as simultaneously merged with, and separated from, the patient.

The self psychologically oriented therapeutic stance is sometimes mistakenly believed to be supportive or sympathetic, as if the therapist is expected to be kind and gratifying, and to substitute in the here-and-now for the deprivation that the patient had suffered in early development. However, it is important to stress that self psychology does not assert that by providing corrective emotional experience in the here-and-now, those past deficits can be repaired or filled in. The therapist's transforming-repairing activity that enables such transformative process involves the therapist's awareness of failures in being empathic to the patient's needs. Provided that the therapist is successful in creating an empathic milieu, these failures will not be harmful. On the contrary, these failures, and the therapist's ability to analyze them in the transference within the basic empathic milieu, are what bring about the transmuting internalization: the process in which the patient (or the child, in normal development) undertakes the functions of the self thus far fulfilled by the therapist or the parent and independently executes them (Kohut, 1971). In other words, this is the process of growing up or being cured.

In infancy and childhood, the child needs to be sympathetically mirrored in the eyes of a parent who looks upon her with joy and delight and provides basic approval. The therapist's task is to create the proper ambiance for mobilizing the patient's demands for mirroring and for the free expression of these demands in the session. Self psychologically informed therapists meet these needs by acknowledging and attempting to understand the patient's feelings, wishes, thoughts and behaviors from the patient's perspective. This is vicarious introspection/empathy. The therapists do not soothe the patient and are not actively enthusiastic about the patient. They understand, justify and interpret the patient's yearning for soothing and confirming responses and acknowledge it. They do not actively admire or approve of the patient's grandiose experiences. Rather, by knowing the crucial role of such experiences in normal development, they can explain to the patient their role in the psychic equilibrium.

Kohut (1984) divides the therapy into two phases: understanding – the empathic mirroring stage; and explaining – the interpretation phase. He suggested that there are patients with severe disturbances of the self with whom the entire therapeutic work can be done in the first phase. For eating-disordered patients, prolonged dwelling in this first stage of empathic mirroring is crucial. These patients have rarely been understood and accepted for what they are and can therefore experience interpretation, particularly at the beginning of therapy, as an imposition of something from without (Bruch, 1985). The unique therapeutic stance of selfobject is especially significant for the therapeutic issue of interpretation experienced from within or from without (Schwaber, 1984).

To fully understand this stance, an explanation of self and selfobject is in order. Self is the center of the individual's psychological universe. It is what we refer to when we say "I feel" such and such, "I do" such and such. The healthy human self is experienced as a sense of wholeness, aliveness and vigor, an independent center of initiative over time and through space. This is the essence of one's psychological being (Tolpin, 1980).

When individual A approaches another individual B and needs and expects B to fulfill A's internal needs that A cannot fulfill for himself or herself, then we can, in self psychology terms, say that A refers to B as a selfobject. A on that occasion expects B to behave as if B were not an independent center of initiative. In other words, the term "selfobject" refers to that dimension of our experience of another person that relates to that person's function of shoring up our self (Kohut, 1984, p. 50).

The internal needs of the self that we have been referring to are needs of self-esteem, regulation of emotions, calming, soothing and a feeling of continuity over time and space. The healthy self can, to a great extent, meet these needs. It can largely regulate self-esteem and it can calm itself. It maintains a sense of continuity, coherence, consistency, cohesiveness and clarity of experience patterns even in the face of considerable stress. In the course of such healthy functioning of the self, others may serve as selfobjects, but the individual relies on them in a mature and limited manner.

Self psychology (Kohut, 1971) asserts that even healthy and mature individuals need their internal needs to be fulfilled, at least partially, by selfobjects. However, their reliance upon such selfobjects is flexible and mature, i.e., they can endure and even outgrow failures of such selfobjects. The unhealthy self, on the other hand, is largely dependent – and sometimes totally and desperately – on selfobjects to do what the underdeveloped self cannot do.

Wolf (1988) illustrates how a toddler may evoke selfobject response from his mother, whereas the same response cannot be expected in the case of an older child. An 18-month toddler throws a ball, hits a vase and smashes it. As long as the mother can be impressed with the athletic achievement, her response is a selfobject response for the child – she is able to share the child's viewpoint and be happy with him. When the mother is angry at the child for smashing the vase, she acts as having independent interests of her own. This example demonstrates that the mother cannot always serve, and should not always serve, as a selfobject for the child. If she provided the child with enough selfobject experiences, an occasional failure and acting as an independent object would lead to the child growing up through the process of transmuting internalization.

In childhood, the healthy emergence of the self depends upon appropriate selfobject experiences. When treating patients with disorders of the self, the therapist renews the growth of the patient's self by serving as a selfobject for the patient. The therapist does that mainly through meeting the patient's need of understanding, acknowledgment and approval of his or her unique perspective. As noted earlier, compared to the traditional therapist, the self psychologically oriented therapist emphasizes more and stays longer in the first stage of therapy – the phase of emphatic understanding – before proceeding onto the explaining stage – the phase of interpretation (Kohut, 1984). The therapist acknowledges the patient's unique perspective, and by interpreting "from within" rather than "from without" (Schwaber, 1984), evokes selfobject experiences in the patient and thus renews the growth of the self. An essential element in this process is the therapist's awareness of potential re-traumatization in the transference caused by inevitable empathy failures. The therapist conveys to the patients his or her special awareness of such recurrent failures by interpreting them to the patient. The therapist's awareness of this rupture and repair allows the therapeutic process to proceed and for internal mechanisms of regulation to be built within the self.

Barth (1991) describes how eating-disordered patients lack the sense of being understood. She describes how much they enjoyed the experience of someone making an active effort to understand their perspective. She vividly describes sessions with such patients, in which whenever the patient felt the therapist's perspective to be discrepant from her own, the patient felt criticized and diminished. As therapy progresses, patient and therapist learn to identify when the therapist is less attuned to the patient's perspective. Patients in advanced stages of therapy can talk about their hurt feelings rather than attempt to restore a sense of self cohesion through bingeing and vomiting (Barth, 1991).

Self psychology views eating disorders as disorders of the self. The core conceptualization of the disorder and its cure is that anorexic and bulimic patients cannot rely on other human beings to fulfill their selfobject needs. Instead of relying on people, they resort to food to fulfill these needs (Barth, 1991; Geist, 1989; Goodsitt, 1985; Sands, 1991). Kohut (1971) essentially described two main selfobject needs: mirroring selfobject needs and idealizing selfobject needs.

The anorexic patient derives her selfobject needs from food mainly through mirroring selfobject experiences. Her need of grandiosity is met not by admiration or approval from other human beings but rather from her own conviction that she possesses supernatural powers that enable her to avoid food. Anyone meeting anorexic patients knows how proud and triumphant they feel whenever they lose another pound. This sense of victory and supernatural or even immortal powers is also apparent in many memoirs written by anorexic patients (Verbin, 2016). Their perceived ability to ignore this substance, food, fulfills mirroring selfobject needs and evokes a great sense of reward, described by one of our patients as being "wonderful, strong, supernatural, above natural powers." This sense of victory is accompanied by satisfaction and self-contentment. It validates the patient's sense of grandiosity (Kohut, 1971).

The bulimic patient satisfies her selfobject needs through food mainly through idealizing selfobject experiences (Barth, 1991; Sands, 1991). She experiences food as an omnipotent power. It provides comfort, soothing and security. It regulates painful emotions like insult, anger, shame, guilt, depression or anxiety (Barth, 1991). Since the eating-disordered patient experiences food and its associated rituals as the main source for fulfilling selfobject needs, she defends it with the same intensity that other people would adhere to a human selfobject.

Goodsitt (1985) identifies in the anorexic patient an extreme manifestation of her inability to refer to human beings in order to fulfill her selfobject needs. She aspires to live as if she is a selfless human being. To ensure such selfless position, she fulfills selfobject needs for others, mainly her parents. Clinging to the position of being a selfobject for others is an effective barrier preventing others from serving as a selfobject for her. Her selflessness is demonstrated through her alienation from her very basic needs, such as nutrition and occupying space in the world. Avoiding occupying space to the extent of almost diminishing one's body is the most extreme expression of selflessness.

A typical saying of many parents of anorexic patients, confirming this observation, is that "she was our best child." "She was obedient and never thought of herself and was always conscientious and aware of the needs of other family members." These observations ensue from the basic position of the anorexic patient as a selfless human being who devotes herself to the fulfillment of others' selfobject needs. The anorexic patient's great feeling of triumph upon losing more and more weight actually signifies that she is looking for ways to gratify her grandiose needs; but the content that stands behind the triumphant feeling is again toward selflessness. This is because she is saying in effect, "I can be admired by my success in relinquishing myself."

Self psychology allows for a therapeutic approach that addresses the anorexic patient's pathological position toward herself. The self psychologically oriented therapist would look for the patient's unique subjective perspective even if this perspective is peculiar or weird. By the very attempt to look for her perspective, the therapist conveys to the patient the sense that someone values her self highly enough to acknowledge and seek. The therapist's behavior provides the patient with an empathic milieu. Namely, according to self psychology, it is not necessarily a warm milieu that is required, but a milieu seeking to understand the individual's subjective perspective. Note that understanding does not necessarily mean agreeing. The individual needs someone who would make an effort to understand his or her perspective, even if that someone disagrees with it. Kohut (1984) asserts that the therapist's understanding and acknowledgment of the patient's possibly pathological perspective is not to be feared as causing the patient to cling and adhere to this perspective. On the contrary, when the patient feels that the therapist understands her perspective, she can harness her powers to examine her own ambivalence toward the pathological perspective and rely on the therapist to grow.

After the anorexic patient feels that her self is bolstered by the therapist's search for it and ability to acknowledge it, she can also accept interpretations as to her selflessness and selfless behavior. It is interesting to note, in this regard, a side note of Kohut (1971) saying that the anorexic patient must nourish her self to live, but her life is in danger for her inability to do so because she cannot think of herself as someone worth nourishing.

Self psychology (Geist, 1989; Goodsitt, 1985; Sands, 1991) suggests that eating disorders originate, like other disorders of the self, from chronic disturbances in empathy of the caretakers in early childhood. Eating disorders are unique in that at some crucial point of development, the disordered girl invents an entire alternative system to fulfill selfobject needs. In this system, distorted eating patterns – either avoiding food or bingeing – are used instead of human beings, and the child relies on them because her previous attempts to gain selfobject responses from her parents were frustrating and disappointing.

Geist (1989) maintains that the underdevelopment of the self is expressed as a severe, malignant sense of emptiness. To defend herself against this sense of emptiness, the eating-disordered patient attempts to monitor and control it through her symptoms. She attempts to gain control over the sense of emptiness through voracious and compulsive eating, or through creating "controlled emptiness" by purging (in bulimia) or by avoiding food (in anorexia). Geist suggests that eating is the activity most closely related to filling up or emptying. Therefore, food can become a reliable selfobject for the eating-disordered patient when she symbolically struggles with a sense of emptiness. Sands (1991) adds another element to explain why food and eating behavior can serve as such an attractive substitute for a human selfobject. Food is the first medium through which experiences of soothing and comfort were provided to the child by parental figures. Ulman and Paul (1989) further suggest that since the bulimic patient does not believe that she deserves to be indulged, her purging activity is her attempt to undo the overindulgence of the binge.

Disordered eating behavior affords the anorexic or bulimic patient a great deal of autonomy over reliance on human selfobject. It provides a certain defense against total fragmentation. However, as Levin (1991) simply puts it, in the context of self psychologically oriented treatment of alcoholics, substance can never adequately fulfill the missing functions of the self. Substance taken in must, obviously, go out. Stable regulators can be built up only through transmuting internalization of self-selfobject relationships with human figures. It is noteworthy in this regard that Kohut (1977a) mentions that in treating a prolonged addiction to drugs or alcohol, it is almost impossible to turn to a human selfobject.

The aim of therapy of eating disorders is to reestablish the confidence in the ability of close interpersonal relationships to mitigate dysphoric states. For the therapist, such an endeavor requires much effort and patience, which in turn requires plenty of time. The basic assumption of self psychology, as accurately put by Sands (1991), is that if therapists provide an empathic milieu and analyses the patient's fear of another re-traumatization in her relationship with the therapist, the archaic narcissistic needs would be harnessed and mobilized toward the therapist in the transference.

In this context, Geist's (1989) distinction between the object relations of borderline personality disorder and eating disorders is highly relevant. Borderline personality disorder patients swing between fury and fantasies of destroying the object, on the one hand, to immense attraction and desire to unite with the object, on the other. Unlike them, eating-disordered patients entirely give up the possibility of relating to human objects as a source of comfort, soothing and security. It appears that Kohut's (1987a) distinction between symbiosis and selfobject relations is useful in distinguishing borderline personality from eating disorders. In symbiosis, the two parties reinforce one another, whereas in self-selfobject relations only one party satisfies the selfobject needs of the other. According to self psychology, the eating-disordered girl's parents have failed to fulfill their daughter's selfobject needs and moreover, used their child to satisfy their own selfobject needs. Therefore, the eating-disordered patient does not expect human beings to fulfill her selfobject needs. Conversely, the future borderline personality patient is involved in childhood in symbiotic and intense relationship with the mother (Mahler, 1975; Masterson, 1976). As a result, as an adult the borderline patient is deeply involved in human (albeit unhealthy) relationships, with great fluctuations between approaching and distancing.

The following clinical vignettes illustrate some of the issues evoked by self psychology in the treatment of anorexia and bulimia

Hardships of Empathy: Empathy When It Is Difficult to Empathize

Many aspects of an anorexic or bulimic patient's behavior are very difficult to empathize with, particularly the destructive parts. How can a therapist empathize with the anorexic patient's great sense of triumph upon losing more and more weight? Indeed, neither the therapist nor a normal parent could, or should, empathize with each and every aspect of the patient's feeling or behavior, but a basic emphatic milieu must be established to enable growth.

One of the therapists of our staff, acknowledging the grandiose need of an anorexic patient, said to her: "For you losing weight is a great achievement, and even a victory. It is a pity that no one else in the world can admire you for that." In a subsequent session, the therapist managed to convey a message of experience-nearness to the patient by mentioning the tension between his responsibility for her health and her own perspective. He succeeded in that through the metaphor of vertigo, telling her:

> You're like a pilot suffering from vertigo, who plummets towards the sea while convinced he is rising to the sky. All of his senses tell him he is correct, and one can easily understand him, but I am in the control tower, warning the pilot that he is falling.

A further example of the difficult challenge facing a therapist wishing to acknowledge the patient's perspective is bombastic manifestations of the patient's grandiose self. A bulimic patient told her therapist: "I'm so talented. My ideas are equivalent to those of the great philosophers. I am the best student in the whole school. I'm more original and skillful than my teachers." She went on complaining that her teachers fail to appreciate her skills and lower her grades over minor mistakes. The therapist commented that she understands the patient's justified wish to be admired and added that it is a pity that teachers are not as efficient in pointing out their students' merits as they are in pointing out the students' shortcomings. The patient went on and said, "there is something outrageous about teachers who are not aware of their students' talents."

Another bulimic patient, a 28-year-old lawyer, already free of symptoms at this phase of the treatment, demonstrated a burst of grandiosity demanding during a legal proceeding that the judge and the opposing lawyer dismiss themselves because of their "incompetence." She was furious for what she felt to be an underestimation of her intellectual merits illustrated by her articulated arguments. The therapist understood that such a grandiose response was a reaction to the lack of confirmation and appreciation from those surrounding her in court. On the one hand, he realized that confronting her with the adverse implications caused by her grandiose self would not be curative. On the other hand, he felt that he could not empathize with her behavior on that occasion. He resolved this dilemma by referring to the tension between what he understood as the patient's need at that particular moment and his perception of reality. He said:

> I am convinced that at that moment you would have liked me to be on your side, like the child coming home after being beaten up or rejected after fighting other children. He needs his mother to be on his side and calm him down, rather than inquire about his part in the fight.

While admitting a potential empathic failure, the therapist points out the discrepancy between the patient's need for his total approval and his perception of the situation and mentions those elements of the patient's behavior that were not to be investigated at the time. The therapist's ability to suspend his or her subjective evaluation in favor of acknowledging the patient's subjectivity is the highest degree of empathy according to Brandchaft and Stolorow (1984), and itself a substantial encouragement for regrowth of the patient's arrested self. The ability to suspend one's own viewpoint to acknowledge and understand the other's point of view can be considered a major factor in fulfilling the selfobject needs of the other.

This response of the therapist seemed to evoke the patient's curiosity, as she said, "specifically it is about my academic merits that I cannot stand criticism or even a lack of admiration." The therapist warmly confirmed this observation and connected it to her childhood circumstances that rendered this area of life particularly vulnerable.

The next vignette is of a mid-20s bulimic patient. At the time, the patient was recovering from her bulimia and for the first time in her life attempted to relate to human beings in the hope that they would fulfill her selfobject needs, rather than seek satisfaction of these needs in disturbed eating patterns. The patient demanded that the therapist adopt her viewpoint and judgments and vociferously condemned his inability to do so. "I want you, I need you to be happy with the emergence of my femininity. I need you to be happy with my new love affair." Noticing the ambivalence of the therapist, she went on to say,

> even though it might seem to you like another dangerous relationship with a married man, I need your approval and your joy about it. Through this relationship, my femininity will flourish and perhaps there will develop in the future a more stable relationship with a man. Right now I don't need your interpretations about my compulsion to repeat the painful abandonments of my father through these relationships.

The therapist knowing, on the one hand, the potential growth experience of this relationship, but recognizing, on the other hand, the destructive elements of this man's questionable intentions, managed to say,

> I do know how important it is for you that I be joyous and approve of this relationship, but I want to be on the side of all your parts; for example, the part of you that also sees the broader picture of this relationship.

She replied, "put aside for a moment that part and join in my happy and flourishing femininity." When the therapist could not fulfill this well-articulated wish of the patient, she said, "it seems to me that you are stuck. Go and get some supervision."

In another case, the therapist failed to empathize with the self needs of her 24-year-old bulimic patient. The patient had devoted all her life to serving as a selfobject for her disturbed mother and for her younger brother. Only in her latest relationship with her boyfriend could the patient enjoy fulfillment of her selfobject needs. But as is the case with many eating-disordered patients who begin to rely on human beings rather than food as providers of selfobject needs, she had related to him in a somewhat bothersome and exaggerated manner. After a period of several months, the boyfriend complained, "I am there for you, but you are not there for me." He claimed that she does not listen to his needs. The therapist, on that occasion, aware of the truthfulness of the boyfriend's claims, pointed out to the patient the reality-testing aspects of her behavior. Perhaps the therapist was eager to keep the relationship of the patient with her boyfriend from being destroyed. But in group supervision, the group and the supervisor alike felt that the patient's self needs required more attention and empathy than the judgment skills of her ego. The therapist, then, in a subsequent session, said, "how painful it is for you to see that even in this relationship in which you just wanted to be cared for and listened to by another, you are also required to listen to his needs."

Counseling parents of anorexic patients and bulimic patients poses a special challenge to the self psychologically informed therapist, who wishes to understand and acknowledge the subjective experiences of the parent. This is a very crucial step because these parents suffer from their own narcissistic deficiencies. Understanding and acknowledging their perspective not only is necessary for handling their deficiencies but also provides them with appropriate modeling for instances when they try to be empathic with their daughters' subjective experiences. Staying, however, with their subjective experience and acknowledging it may make the therapist feel that at least temporarily he or she is doing it at their daughter's expense.

The father of a 16-year-old anorexic girl who is in parent counseling provides a vivid illustration. During the holidays, both his daughter and his wife requested that the three of them take a trip to the countryside. The father, an archaeologist, agreed but suggested that they travel to the hills where the site of his present excavation was located. The daughter insisted upon traveling anywhere but to the excavation site. The father's immediate reaction was fury. The family stayed home in a depressed mood. During the parent counseling session, the father was told that his daughter, apparently, wanted assurance that he would be ready to give up his own interests for the sake of the family's trip. "True, hills are hills everywhere," agreed the therapist with the father's claims, "but your daughter sought proof that you are ready to devote time and interest to her and to the family by putting your work aside." The parent counselor went on to say that perhaps the daughter was able to articulate such a wish because of her therapy. The father seemed to show an understanding of this new way of thinking and looking at things. Then the therapist spoke of how difficult it is for this father to act on what he now understands and perhaps wishes to do for his daughter, namely, to give up, even for a while, his own needs and interests for the sake of fulfilling hers. The parent counselor had known the family history of the father, whose parents had caused him great suffering by constantly ignoring him and his needs. The counselor said, "I know that after so many years of putting aside your interests and your wishes, you cannot afford once again, even temporarily, to put them aside." The father, moved by the therapist's empathy, burst into tears. "Do you believe," he asked, "that this new awareness in me will help me, even to a small extent, to curb my outbursts?" "Not really," answered the therapist, "and certainly not very soon. But when outbursts occur, you will be able to understand what happened and settle things more quickly."

Experience-Near Stance Vs. Experience-Distant Stance

The following vignettes describe a situation in therapy in which the intervention can be regarded as experience-near, namely, experienced by the patient as close to her subjective experience, or experience-distant. Self psychology is strongly in favor of the former (Schwaber, 1984). In the following three vignettes, the therapists found themselves giving interpretations that can be regarded as experience-distant that is, interpretations "from without." In the first case, the female therapist came from a Kleinian background and had only recently gained acquaintance with self psychology. The improvement in her bulimic patient subsequent to her shift in theory was very substantial. The other two therapists (male and female), although holding on to self psychology for quite a while, failed to adhere to it, as we'll see next.

The first vignette is taken from the therapy of a 27-year-old bulimic patient. The patient was telling enthusiastically and with great joy of a new boyfriend who, she had previously thought, was not interested in her, but was now calling and courting her. The therapist intervened and commented upon the patient's way of speaking: "You are talking quickly, like the way you eat. In both cases, you do this in order to cover up deeper feelings of sadness and anger." The patient abruptly stopped her cheerful story about the new boyfriend and a few minutes later burst into tears. Discussing this incident with the supervisor, the therapist explained that she had reached the conclusion about the patient's anger because she, herself, could not trace her own anger and wondered whether it came from the patient through projective identification (a remnant of the therapist's previous Kleinian training). The supervisor commented: "This was interpretation from without. This might be correct, but it is experience-distant. It did not address the subjective experience of the patient and, therefore, it was not an experience-near intervention." After the supervisor and the supervisee had reviewed more cases in which the supervisee failed to intervene in an experience-near manner, her ability to feel and acknowledge the inner experiences of her patients improved markedly, along with a great improvement in the symptoms of the patient. The patient concluded therapy by saying that the greatest improvement for which she is grateful was not only the relief from her symptoms but also the new feeling that she could initiate and trust her own judgment. The patient highlighted this change, namely, her ability to be an independent center of initiative, relying on internal regulating forces, as the crucial change for her. Her intuitive feeling is intriguing, since along with the encouraging improvement of symptoms, the more crucial changes are the emergence of reinforced internal structures that are able to internally provide regulation of painful emotions and an ability to initiate.

The second vignette is from a therapy of a 23-year-old anorexic woman. The patient argued in the session that the progress in her condition and in her life had begun when she started to make notations about her thoughts, her therapy and especially, about her dreams. "Therefore," she went on to claim, "the credit for my improvement is to my notes and not to the therapist." The female therapist interpreted that the patient was competitive and somewhat belligerent. The supervisor thought that this was an unfortunate and painful example of a failure to empathically understand the patient from within her subjective experience. The therapist in this case had interpreted completely "from without," from an experience-distant perspective. The content of the interpretation might have been correct, but what the patient needed, according to self psychology, was to feel her therapist's considerable efforts to empathically understand her "from within." The patient's newly developing capacity to seek, define and understand her own existence and presence should have been approved of and acknowledged. She needed to feel successful and competent by contributing to her own improvement. The proper order for intervention in such a case, according to self psychology, would be to first make the patient feel that the therapist feels and acknowledges what the patient feels – the great sense of discovering one's competence and capacity to understand herself and contribute to her development. The interpretation concerning competitiveness belongs to the level of object relations rather than to self-selfobject relations and should be postponed until the final stages of therapy and raised only if additional material in this level is accumulated.

The third vignette is from a therapy of a 21-year-old bulimic patient, treated by a male therapist. The patient had only recently begun to date men. In her first steps in searching for human beings rather than food to fulfill her selfobject needs, she had gone about it with great intensity. "You need men's attention in a manner that is more than they can or wish to give," said the therapist. The members of the group supervision team felt that although not incorrect, this statement of the therapist seemed to reflect greater empathy on his part toward other people rather than toward his own patient's desperate need to rely on others. The therapist went on to tell his patients that the boyfriends whom she wished to date were the "cream of the crop" of the boys in her environment. He suggested that she was too greedy and had "big eyes." Alternatively, according to self psychology, he should have empathically understood that the patient's subjective experience of weakness led her to look for a man on whose strength and popularity she could rely.

In the fourth case, the therapist's concern for the patient's physical health made her deviate from an experience-near stance. Her deviation, however, was not reflected in an experience-distant interpretation like the former vignettes, but in a surprising question of the therapist about the patient's behavior toward the inpatient unit's staff. The patient, a 20-year-old woman, severely anorexic for five years at the time, finally agreed to therapy after many hesitations. In one session, the therapist explained how hard it was for her, the patient, to give up her illness, which had practically become an identity for her. The therapist also reflected how agonizing the internal struggle was between the tendencies pushing her toward the illness and away from it. The patient seemed grateful for this understanding of the therapist, and in this spirit of aligning with the therapeutic work disclosed that she used to lie frequently to other people. At the same time, she said how nobody understood her and how she could not talk with anyone. The therapist, who knew that the staff received inconsistent information concerning the patient's height, quickly replied: "How did you lie about your height?" Although the question was asked warmly and empathically, the patient immediately withdrew into herself and for days did not return to the therapeutic work in the same sense of cooperation. The therapist explained that she wanted to gain reliable data that would help determine an accurate BMI (body mass index), which in turn would contribute to planning an appropriate nutritional treatment for the severely ill patient. But this wish has diverted the therapist from an experience-near understanding of the patient, telling her, for instance, "you lie to many people because you feel that nobody understands you, and therefore you are forced not to tell the truth because your truth is not understood." It should be stressed that this kind of dilemma, between a therapist's wish to stay close to the patient's experience and her concern for her medical condition and wish to advance the physical therapy, is commonly known to eating disorder therapists. It seems that the therapist in this vignette should have done what Goodsitt (1997) calls "managing of the transference," namely, facilitate the idealization of the patient toward the therapist and ask her, based on their good relationship, to cooperate with the nursing team at this point. In other words, the need to attend to the manipulations this patient probably made concerning her height required a longer and fuller response of the therapist who sees herself as responsible for the patient's physical condition, without surprisingly deviating from the ambience of the session.

Self- Selfobject Relations

During therapy, when patients come to realize that the pattern of their mode of being in the world is as selfless human beings who are trying to fulfill others' selfobject needs, they are typically quite shaken by it. However, their ability to integrate this realization into their personality is very slow and difficult. The intellectual absorption of this understanding does not always coincide with the emotional one.

The patient in the next vignette, a 27-year-old bulimic woman, was already in a very advanced stage of therapy and was symptom free. She had begun mature relationships with other people, both in object relations level and in self-selfobject relations level. Her maturity was reflected in her capacity to rely on her own judgments and preferences as a core directing her life and regulating her mood and self-esteem. Human beings, at this stage of therapy, have become the potential source of filling selfobject needs, and her reliance on them was mature rather than archaic. However, even at such advanced a stage of therapy, she said, "only you" ("you" being plural, perhaps referring to the whole clinic staff)

> have supported what I am, even before I could notice that I am someone. Now it's very strange for me to feel that I can rely on my own judgments and preferences and that I can act for my own benefit and interests and pay no internal price for it. I feel, though, that it is difficult for me to believe that there is a place for me in this world. I understand it in my intellect, but I don't feel it yet and cannot completely believe it.

Another bulimic patient, a 20-year-old woman in the initial phases of therapy, articulated her difficulties in seeing herself as an independent center of initiative.

> How are other people able to reach a decision? I am empty inside. If I want to look inside of me to see what I want, I see just emptiness. I can only fill it with food or with the wishes of others.

An anorexic patient, also a 20-year-old woman, said,

> I am used to looking for and observing what fits the others. If my boyfriend Danny needs me to smile, I smile. I've become an expert in reading facial expressions. Depending on what my sister and my

father need, I will be there to fulfill it. I can spend hours calculating when my brother will use the bathroom and then wait for hours, avoiding occupying the bathroom because he might need it.

At this stage of therapy, the therapist showed the patient that this was a feature of her being; namely, she was trying to be a selfless human being fulfilling others' needs and avoiding taking up space. The patient recalled her father's expression saying, "you developed a rear end" (in Hebrew this phrase connotes a sense of entitlement, high-hatting and a sexual innuendo). He was referring to the feminine curves she started to grow and said it mockingly. She took this double meaning as expressing her father's criticism both of her entitlement to occupy space in the world and feel comfortable about it, and of her sexual development. In the following sessions, she brought up many recollections of places and situations in which she felt extremely uncomfortable with taking up space, like riding a bus. Gradually, her ability to feel comfortable with the space she takes had increased, with first manifestations being her ability to enjoy the space she takes in parties with friends.

Another significant example of a sense of selflessness and existence only to fulfill others' needs may be found in a patient disclosing that she could sing while driving her car only when her son, as a little kid, was riding with her. "It was as if it was just for him, just in his presence, I am allowed to sing. For myself, when I am alone in the car – never." She cannot enjoy relaxing, easy sunbathing or watching TV. She feels that she must work ceaselessly or check and see if her husband needs anything from her, and despite the husband's clear discomfort, she keeps calling him "sir." It is only once a year, in their annual vacation, that she can let herself feel the joy of rest and relaxation.

In one of the sessions, she said, "I have no self-respect." After the therapist showed her how she never occupies space in the world, she told him that she went out very early to work every day so that her car would not add any burden to the heavy morning traffic. When she drives and someone drives behind her she moves away so to not disturb. She never told her colleagues that she held a doctoral degree and used to undertake all cleaning tasks in the lab. When she said, "I always want to be little," the therapist completed her sentence by saying that she wants to be little both mentally and physically through anorexia.

I sit on a beanbag seat to be close to the floor, rather than on a chair like anyone else. When I serve everyone with coffee at home, I obviously serve them with clean cups, but for me I always make coffee in the same dirty cup. It is filthy already, but I still drink from it.

When the therapist inquires for the reason, she says, "I don't know why I do it. I humiliate myself, despise myself with it, and only now I can see it. It is as if I am not worth washing the cup for my own sake."

Another 22-year-old anorexic patient said, "I can either talk or eat. Doing both is occupying too much space in the world." If she found herself talking "too much," she will increase her refraining from eating on that day or at least refrain from eating "healthy food" like tofu as a punishment of taking too much space. In the same vein, a 25-year-old anorexic patient said, "To eat is not to be gentle, not to be weak. I would like to be gentle and weak and by doing so, to open room for other people to take up space. To be weak and sick is to be gentle." She went on to say, "If I don't eat then I am purified because I don't ask anything for myself at the expense of others."

Extreme, almost psychotic, utterances of two patients in the same line of thinking were: "Every breath of mine is at the expense of someone." "Every kilogram of mine is a burden on Earth." I say "almost psychotic" because they immediately say: "Rationally I know this is not so, but I feel it to be."

The next two vignettes are from therapies of girls who only recently began to develop some sense of resistance toward their tendency to devote themselves to fulfilling others' needs. A 19-year-old anorexic girl found herself very much involved in the arrangements required to build two new rooms in her family's house. She frequently mediated between her quarreling parents and encouraged her mother to support her father and help him adjust to his newly developed illness. She performed all these activities from a hospital during the last phases of her hospitalization. Then, in a moment of insight, she asked her therapist and afterwards her parents, "Who is the daughter here and who are the parents? Who is the mother of whom?"

A 19-year-old bulimic patient, after a year in therapy, was struck by a sudden insight into her family's attitudes toward her. Surprised to find that they enjoyed her pattern of fulfilling their needs, she said, "I must have been stupid to sacrifice myself in order to fulfill their needs." She then became very adept at finding incidents in which family members constantly expected her to pay attention to their point of view. She felt that they had automatically included her newly acquired boyfriend into their expectations, namely, expected her to attend to his needs while ignoring her own.

And a third anorexic patient observed, after several months in therapy, how she let her father think, choose and decide for her. She used to go sailing with him in the family's motorboat just because he loved it, while she did not like it at all. When she said "he grew bigger instead of me," she was expressing her self-deprecation, giving up on her own self for the fulfillment of his needs.

The countertransference of a therapist from our team illustrates the feelings aroused in a therapist. This female therapist was in a process of self-selfobject relations with a bulimic girl in the initial and most demanding stages of her ability to expect people to fulfill her selfobject needs. "I feel," said the therapist, "like a programmed robot, when you demand me to make all sorts of phone calls to schedule you doctor appointments." The patient burst angrily into tears: "It is none of my business to know how you feel and you need not disclose your weaknesses to me!" In a subsequent session, the therapist expressed understanding of the patient's need to see her as a strong omnipotent object who can fulfill all her needs. She said: "In your first attempts to trust human beings as providers of your needs, you have perhaps an understandable wish to feel in full control over me as you had over the substance [the food]." Another example of feeling dehumanized by a demand of a bulimic patient to fulfill her selfobject needs was aroused in a male therapist in response to the following statement by his patient: "I need you simply to just to sit here and admire me. I need it very much. I don't want you to do anything else; just sit and admire."

A 23-year-old bulimic patient, a year into therapy, presents a good illustration of the ability of the patient to observe her first attempt to relinquish food and begin to refer to human beings as potential providers of her selfobject needs. At the beginning of therapy, she expressed her attraction to food: "I love food so much that I think I'll never fall in love with anyone." She went on to explain why she prefers a cake to a boyfriend. "With a cake, you don't have to look at its face after you devour it, but a guy, if you want to be with him desperately, you will be embarrassed to look at his face afterwards." With progression of therapy, the patient felt great happiness whenever she chose human beings over food. She was astonished to realize that only the presence of a specific figure, her boyfriend, could totally remove her attraction to bingeing and vomiting. With the beginning of the relationship with this boyfriend, she noticed that his presence, his look, his smell and his touch could overcome all the attractions of food. No other human being, neither her girlfriends nor her family members, had a similar impact on her. "Had I been with him 24 hours a day, I would never binge." In the final stages of therapy, the patient could point out certain sessions and say, "that kind of feeling, being understood, can remove my intentions to binge and vomit."

Concluding Remarks

Self psychology attributes a central therapeutic role to the therapist's efforts to understand and acknowledge the patient's unique perspective. The therapist endeavors to understand even the patient's most bizarre feelings, thoughts and attitudes from within the patient's subjective experience. Such a therapeutic approach has great curative potential for eating disorders in two major respects. First, it conveys to the eating-disordered patient the message that she deserves to have a "self." The fact that someone is making an effort to look for and to understand her viewpoint and is listening to her conveys the sense that she is worthy of having a viewpoint of her own, to have a self that constitutes a center of initiative and choice and to have someone (the therapist) fulfilling for her one of the central dimensions of selfobject, namely, acknowledge and approve her subjectivity. She learns that a human being can serve as a selfobject for her and that she is not obliged to ever be the selfobject of others. The therapist's approach conveys the message that the patient is worthy of the services and efforts of a human selfobject. The patient meets a human being who does not need her as his or her own selfobject, and even empathically analyzes her habits of serving as a selfobject to others. Second, such a therapeutic stance of the therapist may restore in the patient the hope that human beings, rather than the substance she previously used to rely on, can provide her selfobject needs. Only through these self-selfobject relationships with human beings, in contrast with inanimate substance like food, can her self-structure be repaired through the process of transmuting internalization. Namely, the inevitable empathy failures are used for the patient as an opportunity to fulfill for herself what the selfobject could not fulfill in that instance. This process is facilitated by the therapist taking responsibility for his or her failure.

Hilde Bruch, whose pioneering work in the field of eating disorders remains a landmark in the literature, intuitively felt that the two psychoanalytic models of her time – the psychosexual model and the object-relations model – did not fit the treatment of these disorders (Bruch, 1985, 1988). Attempting to summarize her lifelong contribution to the field, she said that the theory of self psychology systematically conceptualizes the clinical phenomena and techniques that she intuitively developed.

Swift (1991) suggests that Bruch's greatest contribution to the field lies in her recommendation to change the therapeutic stance toward the eating-disordered patient. Before the emergence of self psychology,

Bruch emphasized the importance of confirming "the internal reality of the patient" (Bruch, 1970, 1973). She objected to therapists giving interpretations from a "superior position." (Or shall we say, in self psychology terms, "experience-distant"?) She shunned an interpretative approach because she was concerned that interpretation is often experienced by the anorexic patient as a recapitulation of early trauma in which the anorexic patient was told what she thought and felt by a "superior other." She believed that interpretative interventions only confirmed the anorexic patient's sense of inadequacy and they also interfered with her confidence to express herself (Bruch, 1970, 1973). This position evoked Swift's (1991) criticism, arguing that Bruch abandoned the most important psychotherapeutic tool of interpretation. The therapeutic stance as suggested by self psychology may resolve this dispute. According to this approach, interpretations are given only after a long phase in which the patient feels empathically understood, and after she experiences the therapist who gives them not as a distant object but as a selfobject. Thus, the patient will experience interpretations not as something imposed from without but as something given from within.

The self psychological view of symptoms and defenses is another major element that renders self psychology helpful in the treatment of eating disorders. The eating-disordered patient ferociously defends her pathological eating pattern, like someone defending the existence of the self itself. This is because she feels that if she gives up her eating behaviors before genuine selfobject substitutes can be found, she is seriously endangering her self-cohesion. Ornstein (1990) states that the self psychological approach to defenses and symptoms is very different than the confrontational approach adopted by classic psychoanalysis. According to Ornstein, whereas classic psychoanalysis views defenses as obstacles that should be removed layer by layer, self psychology views them as performing the crucial psychological function of protecting a vulnerable self from further depletion or fragmentation.

The eating-disordered patient treated according to self psychology will feel that even her self-defeating and self-destructive behavior patterns, which were thus far the target of condemnations and confrontations, are looked upon respectfully and understandingly as her attempts to restore and maintain a sense of cohesion, wholeness or vigor of the self. This attitude is consistent with the message that the therapist conveys to the patient, that her unique self deserves attention and her archaic needs warrant acknowledgment. Instead of being confronted with her behavior, the behavior is explained to her. She learns that she cannot abandon this behavior until she can rely on human beings to act as potential providers of her selfobject needs, and until inner structures are established to take some of the roles of the external selfobjects.

Sands (1991) vividly describes a case in which the patient was astonished by the understanding attitude of her self psychologically informed therapist who had explained her disturbed eating patterns. The patient asked, "How can you say to a young girl that the Ipecac that she took to bring on vomiting was taken by her as an attempt to feel psychologically better?" The therapist answered, "I'm trying to understand many aspects of your behavior, amongst these, the reasons for your bingeing and vomiting." Her previous therapist viewed those eating-disordered behaviors as suicide attempts. While the destructive nature of those behaviors did not go unnoticed by the therapist, the self psychology therapist did not overlook the curative and restorative (however failing) attempts that these behaviors embodied for the patient. When the patient sees the genuine attempts of the therapist to understand her subjective viewpoint, suspending for a while the judgment of the reality-testing elements of that behavior, she herself will take the next step to recall and remember these elements (Kohut, 1984). Perhaps the patient's puzzled response about the Ipecac is an example of her taking such a step.

Idealization of the therapist is a frequently occurring emotion in patients. Idealization arises partially as a reaction to the great relief and gratitude toward someone who affirms the patient's viewpoint and acknowledges her subjective experience. This emotion originates mostly in the individual's developmental need to have an idealizable figure who can supply calmness and soothing. More often than not, a therapist will find this even more difficult to bear than devaluation. Self psychology warns the therapist against rejecting this developmental need (Kohut, 1968). It objects to the interpretation of such idealization as a defense against other feelings, e.g., aggression, hatred or envy (as Klein (1957) might have interpreted). Sands (1989) even suggests that therapists check on whether patient's devaluations of them are manifestations of their defenses against their long-term unmet needs for idealized selfobjects.

To conclude, the central contributions of self psychology to the treatment of anorexia and bulimia as reviewed in this chapter, are:

1. The therapist's unique position as a selfobject, who attempts to be emphatic to the patient's viewpoint from an experience-near stance.
2. Conceptualization of food (or avoidance thereof) as fulfilling selfobject needs.
3. Recognition of the significance of the symptoms for the patient.

It was suggested in this chapter that self psychology's unique conceptualization of self-selfobject relations, and of resistance and defenses constitutes a therapeutic stance that especially fits the therapeutic needs of eating-disordered patients.

The chapter presents clinical vignettes, which focus on three central issues that illustrate the opportunities and dilemmas advanced by this psychoanalytical development:

1. Maintaining empathy for patient's actions or attitudes toward which the therapist finds it hard to be emphatic.
2. An empathic understanding from within, from an experience-near position, as opposed to an interpretation from without, experience-distant.
3. With progress in therapy, transforming self-selfobject relations with food into self-selfobject relations with human beings.

3 Evidence Basis for Psychodynamic Self Psychology in Eating Disorders

Eytan Bachar

The purpose of the present chapter is to present the empirical basis for the capability of the theory of psychodynamic self psychology to predict in cross-sectional and prospective longitudinal studies, both the development of and the remission from eating disorders. In addition, we present the effectiveness of psychodynamic self psychological treatment in a randomized control study over two other techniques.

The anorexic patient's tendency to relinquish her own interests, give up her well-being, deny even her most basic needs including nourishment and sacrifice herself for the sake of fulfilling others' needs, was described in the two previous chapters. In 2002, we (Bachar et al., 2002) developed the Selflessness Scale to tap and quantify this tendency of the eating-disordered patient. The higher the score on the Selflessness Scale, the higher the tendency of the individual to ignore one's own needs to fulfill the needs of the other.

The following examples are representative of the statements of the Selflessness Scale:

I am willing to sacrifice a lot for the benefit of others.
I usually give in to the will of others.
If the family budget is limited I will give up my part.
If someone is unhappy I will immediately turn to comfort him.
My own enjoyment is the last thing that is important to me.

In 2010, we (Bachar, Gur, Canetti, Berry, & Stein, 2010) found empirical support to the theoretical conceptualization of self psychology, which points to the etiological role of the selflessness position and being selfobject for others in eating disorders. The Selflessness Scale predicted the development of eating disorders in a prospective longitudinal study, over a two- and four-year follow-up. We followed seventh-grade females in a large community-based sample over four years. The Selflessness Scale predicted the development of eating disorders in these participants with a sensitivity of 82 percent, that is, in 82 percent of the cases, the scale predicted correctly that they would develop an eating disorder from the baseline to a two- and four-year follow-up. While a high score on the Selflessness Scale predicted the development of an eating disorder, a normal or lower score on the Selflessness Scale (i.e., when the adolescent did not tend to ignore her own needs and serve the needs of others), served as a protective factor from developing eating disorders, even in an at-risk population (Bachar et al., 2010).

An interesting finding by Bachner-Melman, Zohar, Ebstein, and Bachar (2007) shows that the patient with AN, is "proud" of her selflessness position. They found that the higher the score of selflessness, the higher the tendency of the patient with AN for higher self-esteem, while no such correlation was found in normal controls. Bachner-Melman and colleagues suggest that it is as if the patient with anorexia nervosa is asserting: "I do not deserve to treat myself well, I should be attuned only to the needs of others."

As we have seen in the previous two chapters, self psychology (Geist, 1989; Sands, 1991) assumes that eating disorders originate, like other disturbances of the self, from chronic disturbances in empathy emanating from the caretakers of the growing child. The uniqueness of eating disorders is that at some crucial point in her development, the eating-disordered child, whose crucial selfobject needs were not being met empathically, invents a new restorative system in which disordered eating patterns are used instead of human beings to meet selfobject needs. The child relies on this system because previous attempts to gain selfobject-sustaining responses from caregivers were disappointing and frustrating. We found empirical support to the difficulties of mothers of daughters with AN, to fulfill the expected role of behaving as a selfobject for their daughters (Bachar, Kanyas, Latzer, Bonne, & Lerrer, 2008). We, of course, expect parents to demonstrate the ability to be selfobjects for their offspring and not vice versa. In this study, we found that the selflessness levels of mothers of daughters with AN were significantly lower than the levels found in control mothers of normal adolescents. We also found a very high correlation between a daughter with AN's selflessness scores and mother's signs of depression, hinting at the possibility that when the patient with AN identifies signs of emotional distress in her mother, she increases her tendency to behave as a selfobject for her. No such correlation was found in the control group between normal adolescent girls and their mothers (Bachar et al.,

2008). Yet in contrast with the previously mentioned community-based prospective longitudinal study and forthcoming longitudinal follow-up study, this correlational study (Bachar et al., 2008) should be supported by a prospective longitudinal study for the direction of causality to be corroborated.

We have mentioned the well-known observation that Selvini-Palazzoli (1985) made long ago that children who are prone to develop eating disorders feel guilt whenever they require something for themselves. Our prospective study (Bachar et al., 2010) showed that children who are high in selflessness tended to develop eating disorders within two and four years. Moreover, in Chapter 2, we quoted parents' observations regarding the self-sacrificing behavior of their daughter who later developed an eating disorder. It might well be that children who are afraid "to occupy space in the world" and who do not feel they have the right to exist and to require that their needs be met may not challenge their parents' selfobject skills enough, and not provide opportunities for them to practice those skills sufficiently. The end result may be a reduced capacity to serve as effective selfobjects for their daughters (Bachar, 1998).

Thus far, we reviewed etiological and predisposing factors and showed the empirical support for the ability of self psychological constructs quantified in the Selflessness Scale to predict the development of an eating disorder. Before presenting the therapy and the evidence basis for self psychology in treating eating disorders, we will review cross-sectional as well as prospective studies showing the capacity of the Selflessness Scale to predict remission from eating disorders.

Bachner-Melman and colleagues (2007) found, in a cross-sectional study, that selflessness levels decreased according to levels of remitting from AN. Similarly, Pinus, Canetti, Bonne, and Bachar (2019), in a prospective longitudinal follow-up study of adolescents who were discharged from a day care unit, with an average of five-year follow-up, found that only low selflessness level in admission significantly predicted remission from an eating disorder in follow-up. In contrast, admission level of depression, trait or state anxiety, and initial level of symptomatology (assessed by clinical interview or self-report EAT-26 scale) could not predict remission in follow-up. When Eating Disorders Inventory (EDI) total score was divided into its 11 subscales, only maturity fears (from the 11 subscales of EDI-2) and Selflessness Scale in admission could significantly predict remission at follow-up, but the strength of selflessness was the greatest.

Evidence Basis for Self Psychological Treatment in Eating Disorders

We found empirical support for the efficacy of the self psychological approach in eating disorders compared with two other interventions. We (Bachar, Latzer, Kreitler, & Berry, 1999) compared a self psychological approach to a specific kind of cognitive therapy – cognitive orientation treatment (Kreitler, Bachar, Canetti, Berry, & Bonne, 2003) and a control/nutritional counseling only treatment, without psychological therapy. These interventions were administered over a one-year period. Patients in the two psychological treatments also received nutritional counseling. It is our belief that nutritional counseling, which includes monitoring the symptoms and teaching healthy eating habits, is always necessary. After initial evaluation, patients were randomly assigned to one of the three interventions: self psychological treatment, cognitive orientation treatment and nutritional counseling control group. Self psychological treatment achieved significantly better results than the other two interventions, both in removing the eating disorder symptomatology and in an intrapsychic variable of the cohesion of the self.

These results of the greater inner gains achieved in addition to the alleviation of the symptoms in psychodynamic therapy versus other approaches is consistent with the recently published large randomized controlled study published by the Anorexia Nervosa Treatment of Out-Patients (ANTOP) study, where it was found that the only significant difference among the three approaches – psychodynamic approach, optimized treatment as usual and CBT – was that in the variable of recovery (combined BMI and general eating disorder psychopathology), psychodynamic achieved significantly better results than the optimized treatment as usual, while the CBT fell in between without reaching significance. The ANTOP (Zipfel et al., 2014) study researchers conclude their paper by saying,

> Psychodynamic treatments make interpersonal relationships the major theme. Compared with cognitive behavior therapy they are less directive, induce augmented emotional arousal, and target insight more (vs behavior and cognition). In view of difficulties in the field of autonomy that individuals with AN have, we postulate that these specific aspects of psychodynamic therapy contribute to the positive effects of treatment in this patient group.
>
> (p. 135)

4 Transference, Countertransference and Treatment Management

Eytan Bachar

The therapeutic encounter with an anorexic or bulimic patient is tough and complicated for the patient and therapist alike, at least in its early stages. More often than not, the patient does not enter therapy at her own will. Treatment is forced, at least in the beginning, either by parents' or teachers' pressure or formally by a judicial decision. When the patient is already present in the session, she has difficulties relating to her therapist. As explained earlier in Chapter 2, the patient is cathected in substance – food and surrounding rituals – and finds it hard to approach people. We suggested in Chapter 2 that a therapeutic stance of willingness to serve as a selfobject for the patient, rather than merely an object, may facilitate turning to human objects; however, it takes crucial time in the beginning of therapy until the patient can believe that a human being may fulfill her selfobject needs. The symptoms she developed have created balance and equilibrium in her psychic life, and she will fight hard to preserve them. Symptoms fill her life with meaning, and in extreme cases constitute her entire identity. The main failures in the treatment of anorexia and bulimia may be traced back to these initial weeks of therapy. The patient's refusal to show up for sessions or unsuccessful sessions in the beginning of therapy may doom the patient to dangerous, chronic illness. To put it positively, if the patient and her therapists manage to enter meaningful therapy, with therapeutic connection and alliance, and with the duration of therapy not administratively or technically compromised and nutritional therapy available, then significant improvement would appear, up to remission or recovery, in most of the cases. Evidence is provided in Strober's (1998) longitudinal research and Hoek's (2006) study on patients who adhered to therapy, as well as in the case studies presented in the next part. However, the patients who cannot enter longitudinal studies or can be described in case studies are those patients who showed up for two–three initial sessions and dropped out.

Notably, this encounter is as difficult for the therapist as it is for the anorexic or bulimic patient. The therapist has to meet a patient who, at least in the beginning, hardly wants to meet him or her. This is a patient threatened by the prospect of change and would fight to prevent it. Nonetheless, the therapist acknowledges how crucial these preliminary sessions are and how dangerous it is to drop out at this stage. Moreover, the physical danger adds a concerning ticking time element – seldom present in other kinds of therapy. A highly stressful paradox is thus created for the therapist: on the one hand, the disorder's features require considerable time to establish a therapeutic alliance; on the other hand, the physical situation cries for rapid improvement or stabilization. The presence of such clear and dangerous external reality and the therapist's obligation to report to other parties, such as fellow therapists on the multi-professional team and worried family members, insert complexities and stress that are seldom encountered in other treatments.

To complicate matters further for the therapist, on the one hand, therapists know how crucial therapeutic alliance is for successful therapy (Medina-Pradas, Navarro, López, Grau, & Obiols, 2011; Graves et al., 2017) and on the other hand, they know how difficult it is to establish such an alliance with an anorexic or bulimic patient. Moreover, empirical studies point to the danger of developing negative countertransference specifically in working with eating-disordered patients (Thompson-Brenner, Satir, Franko, & Herzog, 2012).

Once the therapeutic relationship is established and the therapy is taking place, both patient and therapist experience powerful transference and countertransference. If in the beginning the patient cannot relate to the therapist and approach him or her at all, with time she develops selfobject transference and clumsily turns to the therapist as an object. Further down the road, immense dependence and gratitude are present. All these modes of transference evoke intense countertransference reactions in the therapist; starting from a sense of deprecation facing the power of substance (food) as fulfilling selfobject needs for the patient; through experiencing difficulties to continue and serve as selfobject, particularly when the patient addresses him or her like a nonhuman object or a machine; to a grandiose feeling of rescue. Along with these countertransference feelings, the therapist also experiences the anxieties and hardships in the face of a demanding external reality.

One of the ways to help patient and therapist to deal with this entanglement of complexities is to align them with a broader group of "holding" therapists. For the patient, such a holding team may be found in the inpatient unit's professional team, or the outpatient multi-professional team, which includes a nutritionist and often a nurse and a metabolic doctor in addition to the psychotherapist. We'll further see in Chapters 11 and 12 that patients felt the inpatient unit's team to be a sort of home with adult "parents" taking care of them. For the therapist, belonging to professional teams of other therapists may be beneficial on several levels. Two such teams come to mind: first, a multi-professional group of caretakers, including a nutritionist, a nurse and a metabolic doctor to help the case management and overall holding of the case; and second, a psychological working group of psychotherapists that would assist with the case's psychological complexities.

A common mistake of therapists treating anorexic and bulimic patients is the overrating of the patient's ability to take care of her body. The therapist may be illuded by the false self-sufficiency of the patient, who seemingly makes no reason to be concerned about. After several weeks of satisfactory sessions, the therapist may fail to recognize the lack of physical progress or even the presence of temporal decline. A third party outside the transference-countertransference pair, which may sometimes give rise to a collusion ignoring the physical condition, may harness the patient and therapist back to dealing with an emergency physical situation. This third party may be the nutritionist or the metabolic doctor. In this regard, Goodsitt (1997) warns against two opposite poles of the therapist's attitude toward the physical symptoms: under-management or over-management. The former stems from overreliance on introspection and connecting to the patient's perspective and the latter from extrospection and observation from the external reality's point of view.

In some cases, the patient cannot stand any deviation of the therapist from an experience-near stance, in favor of attention to her physical condition. She would not stand any intervention, warning or suggestion relating to her health condition. In such cases, and especially when symptoms are severe, appointing another case manager should be considered, someone other than the therapist. A case manager would set the physical parameters according to which the treatment policy would be determined, such as hospitalization, permission for certain activities and so on. An example for a therapist's struggle whether, at a certain therapeutic moment, she should join the team's efforts fighting for a severe patient's physical condition, can be found in Chapter 2. In that case, the therapist shifted abruptly from her experience-near therapeutic stance to a confrontative and confirmative question, "how did you lie to the staff members about your height?" It was a time of dramatic and consistent weight loss when the patient's height changed from one examination to another, disrupting the calculation of the critical BMI. The therapist felt that the information gained in the session may be helpful for gathering information about the patient's sabotage of the physical treatment. The therapist quickly realized that her sudden switch from the session's regular position to gather this information was wrong and compromised the psychological treatment. The therapist then sensed it would have been better to leave the follow-up of this issue to other members of the multi-professional team. In other cases, however, it is possible and even useful and essential that the therapist act directly as an agent responsible for the physical dimension too, guide and manage meal plans and eating behavior. In such cases, the therapist uses what Goodsitt (1997) terms "managing the transference."

A less direct way to contribute to the multi-professional team's efforts to improve the patient's physical condition is for the therapist to use idealization in certain therapeutic moments when this transference is active. The therapist may ask the patient to eat because of her admiration toward him or her. Clearly, such use must be careful in order not to abuse and erode the idealization transference in such a way that would compromise the psychological treatment.

Sharing responsibility with other team members may help the therapist in additional instances when the external reality intrudes into therapy, instances that are not necessarily related to taking care of the patient's physical condition. For example, it is not uncommon for bulimic patients to have incidents of shoplifting, typically of food. On the immediate behavioral level, it is driven by the need to have large amounts of food for bingeing. On the intrapsychic level, it stems from the patient's distrust that she can get things in a legitimate and appropriate way. We saw in the previous chapters how the bulimic patient undoes her attempts for self-indulgence through her vomiting. Similarly, shoplifting is an attempt for self-indulgence but in the forbidden area – the area of rejection and punishment. Sometimes, when a patient gets into trouble with such theft and turns to her therapist for help, the latter must determine in an extremely complicated dilemma: Is the patient's call for his or her help motivated by primary or secondary gain? The second kind is much more complicated, and perhaps it is unwise to attend to it, since secondary gain is an attempt of the patient to take advantage of her disorder to inappropriately achieve social-environmental gains. Primary gain of the mental disorder, however, demonstrates in its very existence a level of psychic organization intended to prevent fragmentation into a worse level of psychic organization.

Alongside all the advantages outlined earlier of working within a multi-professional team, it should be noted that such work can also bring about conflicts, struggles and even damages because the patient meets several professionals. Sometimes the different attitudes of different

team members and the different levels of relationships respectively created with the patient may lead to disagreements and struggles, even to
the point of compromising treatment. A resonance of such situation can
be found in Chapter 6.

In addition to the assistance and support the therapist may receive
from other members of the multi-professional team, in a complicated
disorder such as eating disorders, the therapist should be able to enjoy
a psychotherapeutic working group. Psychologists tend to bring to such
groups complexities of two levels: intellectual/theoretical complexities
raised while treating anorexic or bulimic patients; and emotional complexities stemming from the nature of transference and countertransference that emerge in therapy of such patients.

The perseverance of the symptom often leads to feeling of despair
on the part of the therapist. In Chapter 6, the therapist relates how she
"ran" to her supervision group because despite what she saw as "beautiful understandings," the patient continued to lose weight. The therapist
needed the supervision group to contain her anxiety and enable her to
keep on doing her work with patience and persistence. Inversely, in
Chapter 17, the therapist tells us how her supervision group helped her
to see, when she was desperate, that in fact the patient was considerably improving on the symptom level, while the therapist was preoccupied with her own disappointment of the lack of sufficient intrapsychic
progress, in her opinion. An immense empirical support that a group
supervision can supply to psychotherapists can be found in Franko and
Rolfe's study (1996), in which more than 90 percent of their 71 psychotherapist participants said that sharing experiences in the group supervision was the most beneficial tool in their work.

Considerable emotional difficulties for therapists emerge when the
patients refer to them as if they weren't human beings. So did the therapist in Chapter 7, when the patient told her, "Sit down and admire me.
I am here not like in the presence of a therapist but like in the presence of a journal to write in." Or the therapist in Chapter 2 who said to
her patient, "I feel like a programmed robot, when you demand me to
make all sorts of phone calls to schedule your doctor appointments."
Understanding that such situations occur because the patient refers to
the therapist not as an individual object but as a selfobject would have
made it easier for the therapist. Such a behavior is intensified when
the patient takes the first steps in turning to people to potentially fulfill her selfobject needs after having previously turned exclusively to
substance. We saw in Chapter 2 and we'll see in Chapter 17 that focusing too early on an interpretation of transference as referring to object
rather than selfobject transference, halted the progress in therapy. In

Chapter 2, we saw the therapist's interpretation that a patient's behavior was competitive, an interpretation that was perceived as inappropriate since it focused on object-relation transference (hence the potential competition between objects), rather than transference referring to a selfobject who is not a distinct object and therefore shares the patient's sense of success.

Siding with the self rather than with the ego often requires an emotional effort on the part of the therapist. We have seen in the second chapter examples of therapists who tended to support the advancement of their patient's judgment skills, particularly when the patients were inclined to get into trouble or harm their relationships with others, while it was their selfobject needs that required the therapist's validation more urgently. Further down the road, after the patient's self was improved, the therapist can reinforce the patient's judgment skills when, for example, the patient says, "If I take one bite of food I will never stop eating until I'll blow up." The therapist may explain on such occasion that although this was the patient's fear at the beginning of therapy, now, when she developed inner capabilities of self-direction, self-control and self-restraint, there is no such risk that she'd lose control over her eating. In the eleventh chapter, the therapist tells her patient clearly, even somewhat blatantly, that she can let go of the food measuring ritual since her mental and physical health condition no longer requires such rituals. Obviously, the therapist must constantly check herself to make sure she does not say such things out of impatience but out of careful clinical and therapeutic evaluation.

Activism on the therapist's part as presented earlier is required not only through those references to the importance of the symptoms or the possibility of abandoning them, but in particular at the beginning of therapy to overcome the patient's difficulty to enter a dialogue. Patients with eating disorders often manifest alexithymia, i.e., difficulty to express emotions. They therefore feel tremendous stress when they sense the burden of talking in the session. The therapist must directly and actively encourage the patient to talk: "I know that it isn't easy for you to say what you feel and what passes through your mind. Take your time, and when a trace of thought gains words and you articulate them, say them to me." It is not recommended to enable too long silences at the beginning of therapy, and the therapist, along the same therapeutic line, may say: "When you feel like it let me know what passes through your mind, and don't be embarrassed or hesitate to break the silence."

A therapist working with an anorexic or bulimic patient who has persistently worked in therapy along all stages would feel the dramatic change she undergoes. The therapist would switch from the sense of

taking care of someone fragile, who has troubles to relate to the therapist and to express herself, to the sense of someone who chooses life,
who dares to take up space and who turns to human beings as a source
of relatedness and soothing. The manner in which the patient relates
to her therapist clearly undergoes parallel changes and progress, from
complete lack of relating to the therapist to a clumsy approach to her as
a non-human selfobject. From that point, a greater ability of separation
is created within a relationship that is still filled with a mixture of self
and selfobject, until at the end of therapy the patient is better able to see
the therapist as an independent object.

A fine distinction in the patient's concern for her therapist may illustrate the mental development she had undergone throughout therapy.
Whereas at the beginning, it is common for her to have concern for her
therapist out of the familiar position of serving as a selfobject to others, toward the end of therapy, the therapist is called upon to accurately
diagnose whether the patient's attentiveness to her originates from a
more mature position, that is, a mature concern for a separate and independent object, the same concern referred to by Winnicott in his paper
"The Capacity for Concern" (Winnicott, 1965a).

Part II
Case Studies

5   I Wanted to Disappear

Eytan Bachar

Dana was referred to me for biweekly therapy during the final weeks of her hospitalization in the ward for eating disorders. A 17-year-old pleasant young girl, slender and short stature, she suffered from restrictive anorexia and major depression.

It became apparent in our first sessions that Dana possessed great curiosity about the process of psychotherapy and, unlike the average anorexic patient, desired to express herself and to utilize introspection.

Dana is the oldest child in her family and has three siblings. Dana's father is a carpenter who manufactures both utility items and art materials. Her mother is a college lecturer. At the age of 15, Dana developed the first signs of depression that was seen at the time as a reaction to the loss of her beloved grandmother. At the age of 16, the restrictive anorexia appeared. Her weight decreased until she reached a BMI that was less than 14.

In the initial meetings, it was already possible to see that it was important to Dana to be a "good patient," to impress and to please me. She was aware of this and even made it explicit that it was very important to her to demonstrate that she was interesting and thought deeply so that I would want to treat her. When I inquired whether this was familiar to her from other relationships, she spoke of her mother. Especially as a child, but also as a teenager, she was concerned as to whether she was intelligent enough to be a good conversation partner for her mother. As the therapy progressed, it became apparent that not only was it important to Dana to be interesting enough to her mother, but even more so to fulfill the task she had set herself to calm her mother down and to make her happy. Dana described her mother as forever despondent about life. She remembered how as a small child at the age of four and five, she would see her mother cry and feel the responsibility to go up to her and hug her. If she felt that she had disturbed her mother or if her mother made a comment, even a simple everyday comment like:

"Enough, Dana, wait a minute," she would shrink, withdraw into herself with a bad feeling that she had bothered her mother, that she was not a good child.

Dana attributed the depression she suffered at 15 to an unhealthy relationship she had with a boy in her class who wanted to have sex with her. She acquiesced even though she had no interest in sexual relations and found the experience painful and disturbing. She said she did it for him, so that he would feel enjoyment and satisfaction. "If I can cause someone to feel enjoyment, I will comply even if it hurts me physically or even psychologically."

In the first time she spoke about a dream she brought to a session, she said she dreamt that her parents wanted her to die. She interpreted the dream as representing her anger at her parents who had not prevented the deterioration of her condition that led to her hospitalization. I said that maybe she felt that they had not granted her the right to exist. She did not show up for the next two sessions, reporting that she was ill. When she returned, I asked whether the intensity of the dream or my interpretations about it were intimidating. She considered what I had said but did not agree.

In the following sessions, the theme of her desire to be an interesting discussion partner for her mother recurred. She remembered many instances of feeling the obligation to respond wisely enough to things her mother told her so that the conversation would continue. She felt an obligation to make an effort and not to be simply spontaneous or "natural." I said that she did not believe that anyone would want her if she did not make an effort. "You do not believe that you have the right to exist on your own terms if you do not make an effort to be there for the other." She replied to these interpretations by saying that even here in the therapy, she was not sure that I would want her as a patient unless she made an effort, unless she was interesting and did not bore me.

In the following therapeutic hours, Dana amazed me with her statements: "I wanted to minimize myself by means of the anorexia, to disappear, to starve myself because I had no right to exist. I am not worthy of living." It was clear to both of us that the words "I am not worthy of living" represented something enormous and deep. She said, "I feel that I am a burden to my mother," but when I asked her what she meant, in what way was she a burden, she could only say something that appeared superficial to both of us: "I don't know, maybe I am a difficult child, struggling with my studies."

At this stage, about five months after the beginning of therapy, she began to open up to the world: to be more interested in others, to hang out in town with friends as befits young people, to begin to seek meaning-ful relationships with young men, to complete her matriculation exams and to apply for an elite program in the army, which would require her to fill a valuable and complex educational position. During this period, she showed for the first time a heightened awareness of everyday exam-ples of her self-negation and tendency to serve the needs of others. She related, for example, how she used to forgo her pocket money in order for her brother to receive more, "because he needed more for his pleas-ure outings than I do." Her parents saw this as an example of her gener-ous nature, but at this stage of the therapy she already began to be angry with herself about this behavior pattern. Immediately after she spoke of this generosity to her brother, she remembered an episode when she was about eight years old. She was trying to fall asleep and wanted her parents to come to her bedside. She called them but they were busy talking to an architect about renovating their home. When we attempted to understand why this memory arose at that point of the session, we thought that maybe it came to show her pain that she could perceive another's needs but her parents could not perceive hers. This memory came up a number of times. I thought of it as a *telescoping memory*, that is, an enlarged memory of a single event that probably represented other similar events. That time brought many signs of a budding ability to change the patterns of self-negation and attunement to the needs of others. One example out of many occurred when a friend from the time of the hospitalization asked to stay with Dana and her family over the holiday season.

Dana and her family had planned a pleasurable picnic and hike, and Dana felt that the friend's visit would be a burden for her, especially because of the friend's tendency to share her sorrows and expect empa-thy and support from Dana. "I want to enjoy myself, to worry about myself and not to have to be there for her." She found a compromise solution in not refusing the visit but inviting the friend to only part of the picnic in the hope of not having to devote all her time and energy to supporting her.

In the following months, Dana gained weight gradually and appropri-ately. The eating disorder symptoms became scarcer. She told me that "one can see that my hips are rounder and my bust is bigger." As she also reported several times during these weeks of therapy that she had skipped her intermediary meals, I asked her if these physical changes frightened her and therefore she had skipped the meals. She answered immediately and with great confidence (so much so that I was surprised by the strength of her conviction) that she was happy and wanted to be feminine and sexually attractive. Her developing relationships with the opposite sex proved this. However, despite her desire for intimate relationships and despite her increasing urge to stop with the behavior pattern of denying herself in favor of others, each time she was about to begin a relationship with a new partner she made sure that none of her girlfriends wanted him and if she thought someone did, she declined the opportunity and enabled her girlfriend to initiate the relationship. At this time, with reference to her relationship with her mother, it was very apparent that she wanted to stop feeling so responsible for her mother's well-being. She even made statements like "she should manage her own affairs," and "I definitely will not give up my dates with friends to stay at home with her." However, she immediately felt that it was really difficult for her to do this. She said: "I feel that this task of stopping to feel responsible for my mother's welfare is a good and appropriate plan, but the actualization is far off and I will get there at my own speed."

I had confidence in Dana that "her own speed" of forgoing the pattern of self-negation and of believing in her right to flourish was definitely satisfactory. Indeed, from this time and till the end of the therapy she advanced, albeit with ups and downs, in terms of her occupational and social achievements. An example of her increasing ability to stand up for her rights and demand her space can be seen in an incident that occurred with the supervisor in charge of her in the army. The supervisor used Dana's idea in some lesson but gave the credit for it to someone else. Dana described to me the process she underwent for almost a week as a result of this episode. At first, she was amazed by his giving credit to someone else. She went around for a few days accompanied by a feeling of insult and hurt. The feeling of insult was replaced by great anger that she desired to vent. The first thing she thought of was to binge or to fast seriously, or alternatively to indulge in some heavy sporting activity. But then she decided to free herself of the difficult feelings by relating directly to the person who hurt her. She sat down and wrote a very long email and sent it to her supervisor. She told him that he had made an error in the attribution of credit for her idea, that she was hurt by this and that she wanted him to know about her feelings. I complimented her profusely on the step that she had made. I pointed out that in the past, she had become used to giving up on her place for others and here she could not bear that she was not seen or acknowledged. I complimented her on choosing the more complex and healthy path of directly confronting the person who had hurt her feelings, instead of the simpler and more usual way of coping she would have chosen during her illness, of turning to food, bingeing or starving, to find an outlet for her emotions. In response to my reaction she said:

> In those days I felt that one can feel held through food. When one is fasting or bingeing they can feel something strong physically, as I said, like the feeling of being held, sometimes even being hugged and then you don't need people to rely on.

I thought to myself that she succeeded in her idiosyncratic idiom to express the function of the food via its consumption or avoidance to fulfill selfobject needs instead of human beings.

It seemed that Dana's increased openness to the world and her greater pleasure in her femininity encouraged many young men to make romantic approaches to her. In this field, she demanded of me great precision in every interpretation. She was vigilant in checking that I understood and agreed with the steps she took. "Why does it seem to me that you think that the relationship with such and such boy is good or bad? Why do I think that you think that the connection is too fast or too slow?" She was especially angry if she thought that I was doubtful about the appropriateness of some relationship or another. In addition, her pleasure in her body and her attractiveness underwent fluctuations. On the one hand, she was very proud of her attractive body and enjoyed appearing in a bikini. On the other hand, she felt shame and was uncomfortable with feeling proud of her body and sexual attractiveness. I interpreted to her that she still did not completely believe in herself and that it was new to her to feel that it was permissible for her to flourish, to enjoy and to succeed. Associated with these insights were dreams in which her cousins, who were boys of her age, appeared to oppose her development as a woman. While she continued to demand, almost until the end of the therapy, that I express my opinion about her relationships with men, she typically complained about the accuracy of my perceptions: "You don't understand precisely."

In some of the cases, she proposed ideas about this or that boy that appeared to me to be much more accurate than my understanding. This ability of hers to grow and to succeed in interpreting herself can be understood in terms of "transmuting internalizations" (Kohut, 1977b) i.e., the ability to grow when the caretaker (in this case the therapist) fails to fulfill all the individual needs but still generally supplies an understanding environment.

A year after the beginning of the therapy, the central theme turned to her relationship with her father. It is to be noted that according to Kohut (1979), after treating the injured self, the strengthened self in many cases enables the Oedipal conflict to come to the surface (a similar phenomenon can be observed in Chapter 16). This step of working through the relationship with her father began with a dream in which a large "sensual hairy figure" was trying to seduce her. During the associations of the dream, I asked if it was possible that the figure could be her father. She agreed with embarrassment that it was true, that she wanted to say so but was ashamed. In this session, and every few sessions for some months after, the subject of her relationship with her father arose. In the beginning, she wondered if the fact that she was not always fully dressed when at home could arouse her father. As if he had read her thoughts, her father told her that her state of undress disturbed him and could also possibly arouse her younger teenage brother. She answered him angrily and asked why he did not think that his state of undress aroused her. Following this, she dreamt a number of dreams in which she engaged in sexual activity with her father. In those sessions, she described behavior and traits of her father of which she had not been aware of previously. In her eyes and in the eyes of others, he was perceived as sensual, very handsome and sexually attractive. She even suspected that he was sexually active outside of home.

I said that because in the therapy in the last few months, she had been opening up to her sexuality and the possibility of feeling arousal in her body, which was becoming more womanly, she was beginning to desire relationships with men. The fact that her father was an attractive, sensuous man who was possibly sexually active with other women besides her mother caused her to dream of being sexually attracted to him.

During the time when we were working on the relationship with her father, her overt behavior toward him was belligerent, removed and rejecting. With the progress in the work on the Oedipal issues she could better understand, with the help of my interpretations, the complexity of her feelings on the one side, but also their normative nature, resulting with the relationship with her father calming down, becoming more quiet, comfortable, mature and even friendlier than ever before. It is possible to see the conclusion of this phase in the therapy in a letter that she wrote to him in which she told him that he was very dear to her, that she was worried about him and that she begged him to avoid self-destructive behaviors like overeating and smoking.

At the same time as the therapy was focusing on the relationship with Dana's father, she had quite a few relationships with young men. However, there was an older man with whom she had a relationship that I deemed not at all healthy. He was a violent man (if not directly toward her), borderline delinquent, always toting a weapon. She detected my doubts about the relationship and responded with much anger: "You are square, inflexible, stuck in your perceptions and don't budge from them." A central element in my interpretations about her relationship with this man was that she sought an illicit, problematic relationship with an older man who was sensuous and stormy, to afford a concretization of her thoughts and emotions concerning her father. As her relationship with her father became more relaxed, mature and friendly, as was apparent in the letter she wrote to him, so the relationship with this man drew to a close. Shortly thereafter, she began a good and stable relationship with a suitable and positive young man, a relationship that continued after the therapy had ended.

It can be surmised that the work that was done on the Oedipal complex, which became possible after months of work on the injured self, contributed to Dana's ability to establish a mature relationship.

One particular session that dealt with that problematic boyfriend is worth mentioning here because of an interesting reaction of hers to my reflections. She told me how she's hiding from her friends and parents behaviors and utterances of that man that were especially inappropriate or even disgusting toward her. I felt how much she was alert, anxious and on guard to any possible unpleasant reaction toward him that I or the environment might have. I felt on that occasion that he is very precious to her and that she is very devoted to protecting him with all her power. I said, "There are nice things in your attitude and it is moving to see how you protect a person who is so dear to you. It is moving and impressive how you defend him."

Suddenly, she burst into tears. I asked her what happened, and she said:

> I am not used to having someone that can connect to my feelings and understand me, even if he doesn't agree with me. I know your opinion of this guy and that this relationship isn't good for me, but still you can see it from my perspective.

Once again, I was amazed by the accurate and delicate ability of hers to express in her own words the importance of one of the basic functions of selfobjects, namely, to suspend one's own perspective in order to connect to the perspective of the needed self.

The strengthening of Dana's own self can also be seen in in the development of her relationship with me. In the first months of the therapy, it was very noticeable that she desired to please me, was concerned that she was taking up space that was meant for others, that she was boring me and that she needed to make an effort to bring subject matter that would interest me. It was as if she almost reached the level of selfobject for me, inquiring almost obsessively as to whether I was insulted by her or disappointed and hurt by her if she did not accept my interpretations. With the growing cohesiveness of her own self, I began to feel that she was beginning to feel and to function in a more equal fashion and to demonstrate her presence in my company. She began to ask me personal questions as if she saw me as an independent object, and she deliberated on whether she should call me by my first name or by my surname and title. She wanted to clarify whether I was too formal or not in relation to her:

> On the one hand, one can see you are working according to some method, one can see you have a method in your head. You are so strict about times and payment. But if you were only strict and formal I could not be here.

Comments like this indicate to me her ability to enter into more equal and mature relationships, to define what she wanted of me. She also said in a very definite and appropriate way:

> You do not allow me to take care of you, like my mother or even my father sometimes expect that I will take care of them. I can actually feel how you are aware of this and prevent me from behaving in that way towards you.

In the last six months of the two-yearlong therapy, we began to prepare for termination. During the last year of the therapy, Dana was free of symptoms. Her BMI was normal, her eating patterns were healthy, organized and balanced. The purging and cutting, which were anyway never frequent, disappeared completely. Dana was very pleased with the success of the therapy. It was apparent how happy she was with her success with men and how she enjoyed their pursuit of her. She was also aware of her success in freeing herself of her enormous awareness of the needs of others: "I used to be so aware of every small movement my mother made with her leg, asking myself whether it meant that she was tense." She was aware and happy about her development, but occasionally there were short bouts of symptoms. I interpreted these short-term "failures" as her difficulty in believing that she was allowed to recover, to flourish, to succeed and enjoy life. At first, she was surprised by this interpretation but later accepted it gladly by saying, "It is really like a new toy for me, that I can be happy, be light-hearted, enjoy life and grow."

Ten years after the termination of therapy, Dana approached me when she saw me in the corridors of the university. We sat down to converse and she told me with joy that she had had no symptoms for years. She was studying and working and was in a good long-term relationship.

In looking back at the therapy with the question on what were the factors that enabled the process to be successful, there are, of course, a number of possible answers and many factors: good chemistry that we had the fortune to experience with each other, empathy, a long period of the therapist being in the experience-near stance, and the perception from "within," from her perspective and not from "without." All of these were definitely present; however, it seems to me, over and above them was her inquiring mind that asked: "Why did I develop anorexia?" After she expressed the thought that "with the anorexia I wanted to make myself small, to disappear, to starve myself because I was not worthy of existing, of living. Living, I am not worthy enough of living," she was able to hold on to the path we found together to free herself of the pattern of sacrificing herself for the needs of others. She began to negotiate this path; first with hesitation, sometimes with feelings of guilt and remorse that she was thinking of herself, but further down the line also with determination and strength and even joy that she is successful and flourishing. Her ability to free herself of the pattern of total attunement to her mother's moods and needs gave her the encouragement and momentum to do this in other aspects of the therapy and in other relationships in her life.

6 Would Sheryl Be Able to Take Up Space?

Michal Man

I first met Sheryl when she voluntarily committed herself to the psychiatric ward at Hadassah Medical Center in Jerusalem. She was 27, intelligent, pleasant and quiet and frighteningly thin. Her blond hair fell on her pale face and hid her big black eyes. She was dressed in cast off, almost sloppy, clothes. At the time of admission, she weighed 34kg (height 1.66m), and her physical condition was poor. She was diagnosed with anorexia nervosa bingeing-purging type. The individual therapy described later was a part of a comprehensive treatment plan, including nutritional and medical treatment, and during her time at the inpatient ward – family therapy.

Sheryl was the youngest daughter after three brothers and two sisters. As a child in a community village, she used to cling to her mother and had difficulties separating from her. Until her sixth grade, she suffered childhood diseases – shortness of breath and severe ear infections. In a family where physical contact was considered taboo and emotions were not communicated, times of illness were the only opportunities to earn some warmth and tenderness from her mother.

At home Sheryl was pseudo-independent, stubborn and was admired for being strong and courageous – the prettiest girl and nothing could stand in her way. At the regional school, however, she was quiet, reserved and preoccupied with her popularity and comparison to others.

Sheryl's sexual development entailed shame and secrecy. In the seventh grade, she went on a diet, and in the eighth grade, she led the girls to compete with each other on who would eat less, for which she was expelled from school. Her poor physical condition went on in high school. Many of her peers sought her company but were rejected. Later on, her bulimic sister taught her how to vomit. Sheryl went on to fasting during weekdays and to binge eating on the weekends. She stopped menstruating regularly in tenth grade. She approached several therapists to treat her eating disorder but did not establish meaningful relations with any of them.

Sheryl served in the army as a clerk, a position to which she was totally dedicated: she prepared feasts for the soldiers and ran the military local convenience store. The soldiers came to know her as the one who did not eat. After a while, she began to secretly eat and vomit. She found herself taking candies from the store, opening packages that were sent to the soldiers and ecstatically searching for food in the staff ward, all while feeling awful humiliation and shame and a constant sense that "everybody knows."

Toward the end of her military service, she had a first and brief contact with a boyfriend. After she was discharged from the army, she moved to Jerusalem and started therapy. To finance therapy by herself, she worked day and night, mainly as a waitress. She did not eat, and on weekends at home, she ate and vomited.

During that therapy, which spanned over a year, her condition further deteriorated. She vomited regularly and used laxatives and even enemas daily. She committed herself in a psychiatric ward for two months, where she gained five kg and continued her follow-up for another year weighing 48 kg. At the beginning, she was happy. She studied art and maintained a rigid regime of therapy and strict meal plans. But the therapists did not know that she was taking obsessive walks an hour after each meal, and binge eating was quick to follow. Therapy was terminated due to the therapists' leaving. Sheryl moved to a rented apartment in town, quit her art studies and started preparatory course to complete her matriculation exams. Again, she was working crazily to gain financial independence and barely graduated from the preparatory course. She looked for a job with children, hoping to regain "the sparkle of life," but when she finally attained such a job, she found herself mainly engaged in cooking for them. She kept herself constantly busy but gradually lost interest in all spheres of life. She also kept moving from one residence to another, hoping for a fresh start time after time. After uncontrollably losing weight, Sheryl started her current therapy by referring herself to Hadassah's psychiatric ward.

The family dynamic was complicated. Sheryl's father was a farmer, practical and alienated from emotions, who lived by strict standards of a lone wolf. Emigrating from North America to Israel by himself at the age of 15, he was not a man of words and communication with him was confusing. Sheryl admired him. She was preoccupied in guessing the message of his eyes and did everything to turn his look from disappointed and degrading to warm and proud. Around the age of ten, she decided to be just like her father and brothers – tough, dominant, in need of no one, a "strong minded" individual.

Sheryl's mother grew up in Israel in a bereaved family, after her older brother was killed in an accident when she was eight. She felt relieved by his death since he used to abuse her. At a very young age, she was sent to a boarding school because her mother (Sheryl's grandmother) had drowned in pathological grief and was not available for her remaining living children.

Sheryl had conflicting experiences with her mother, ranging from enmeshment to stark separateness. In Sheryl's experience, instead of dedicating and sacrificing herself for the family, her mother was in fact busy with her own needs. Sheryl, who did anything to satisfy her mother, grew up feeling that she would never succeed in this task. At the end of an exhausting laborious day at the farm, her mother gave her the feeling that she could go on working; and when she was complimenting Sheryl, Sheryl heard a false tone in her voice.

Since her early adolescence, Sheryl had felt inside her "a block of anger" toward her mother: she would fail to keep her promises; would disclose communications told her in secrecy and would often cut corners; she would act friendly and warmly on the outside, but lacked any true joy with people. All this made Sheryl repelled by the laugh of her mother, up to the point that she stopped laughing herself. The mother signals lack of control for her: Whenever she's upset – she eats and then she is unhappy with her looks; when you tell her a secret – it is never kept. Sheryl swears not to be like her. At the same time, though, she is attuned to her mother's tremendous vulnerability and to the great burden farm labor puts on her, and she volunteers to take her role as a victim.

Despite her efforts, Sheryl's parents did not listen to her or sensed her, and it was like "talking to the walls." They never knew how to limit her help with the labor at the farm according to her strength as a child or when she needed time for her studies. They denied her illness and opened their worried eyes only when her condition worsened.

The family home was characterized by duality: on the outside, the father is strong and assertive and the mother cheerful and friendly; on the inside, they are fragile, vulnerable parents, who are helpless because mourning, separation and guilt dwell in the seemingly happy home. The children also get double messages: on the outside, independence is valued and encouraged, but on the inside, a tight grip is imposed; on the outside, the material generosity is endless, yet calculation is being made behind one's back. The father adores Sheryl for her strength and dominance and at the same time implicitly signals her never to dare to grow up or take up space.

The fact that her parents never explicitly asked for anything only reinforced Sheryl's preoccupation with deciphering their signals and attempting to protect them. Any separation entailed a sense of betrayal, guilt and remorse. Wherever she was, home called her to return but the moment she passed the doorstep back in, she felt the fall of emptiness.

Sheryl's therapy began with a ten-week inpatient admission. It then continued at the outpatient unit twice a week for 11 months.

At the inpatient ward, Sheryl manifests classic anorexic eating behaviors and considerable compulsiveness. She arouses curiosity and admiration among the other patients but rejects any attempt to approach her. The psychiatrist and the social worker functioned as case managers and their behavioral approach easily leads them to power struggles with her. She experiences them as seeing only her "sick part," and the relationship with them is filled with mutual anger.

The nutritionist, the nurse and myself incline toward a softer approach, to partially see Sheryl's healthier parts. Sheryl's internal split between health and sickness, control and ineffectiveness, intrusiveness and neglect is thus being externalized. In a nervous and stubborn voice, she brings to our sessions a sense of suffocation by the limits forced upon her freedom to move and to eat. As her therapist, I walk a tight rope between the treatment plan and between my empathy to her inability to trust the staff members and her unrealistic wish to engage in activities far beyond her physical strengths.

Sheryl is constantly preoccupied with reading others' glances. Despite her efforts, the doctor's facial expression was experienced as derogatory, and this opened the door to working through her relationship with her father. All along the years, she had read in her father's look pain and exhaustion. She fantasized that he suffered from her mother's loudness and disloyalty and volunteered to make it up to him. But she never felt confident that he was proud of her, and during her admission, she felt his devaluation. I mirror her massive preoccupation with deciphering the looks and opinions of others. This preoccupation is burdensome, confusing and mainly leaves no room for listening to herself.

On the other hand, absent any cohesive and distinct self, Sheryl sets rigid boundaries between herself and others, fearing crossing boundaries and thereby losing her own self or the other. At the hospital, she depends on others for provision of goods from outside the hospital, and it raises a tremendous difficulty to ask for them. Behind the ideology she absorbed from her father – never ask anyone for anything – we discover her fear that she would exaggerate and be rejected, along with the fear to coerce the other to act, which would make her feel guilty and obliged.

The intensity of her neediness, the fear of disappointment and of the destruction caused by her fury make her pseudo-self-sufficient. It is only through her disorder that she can outcry her yearning for care and holding and express her anger for their absence.

The metaphor of a snail became our code – a snail folding into its hard shell and declaring it can be on its own. Deep inside it yearns to let go of its snailish uniqueness, but at the same time afraid to be "like anyone else," to be left unattended and to disappear. The big, brown worn jacket in which Sheryl covered herself throughout the entire admission period symbolized this snail. She signaled everyone to leave her alone and at the same time was afraid to take the jacket down so someone might notice she was not thin and sick enough to justify being taken care of.

Sheryl does not risk getting close to me. She defines our relationship as "solely therapeutic" and resists being engaged in the transference. Although she says that our sessions are the only place in which she feels understood, most of the work remains intellectual, with a sense of urgency to "get the work done" and emotional distance. When she cries in my presence, she feels disgusted by herself. I am often pushed to intellectualization and wonder how I can reach her.

Sheryl tells me about her experience of dissociation. She observes herself from without like watching a movie, and sometimes she also does that in the session. When she was in a relationship with a boyfriend, she spoke like from a written script, felt nothing, and only after they broke up she mourned for days. Similarly, the relationships she forms in the hospital seem to pass near her rather than touch her.

In general, Sheryl had difficulty identifying her feelings. Her descriptions were somatic and primary: "A black metastatic lump stuck in the throat like cancer." Later on, she gets less concrete and describes her feelings as "the frozen and paralyzing part." When she is not allowed to freeze her Ensure drink (a calorie-rich drink prescribed, among others, to anorexic patients) and carve the ice for hours instead of drinking it in the liquid form, she feels: "I am being totally emptied." It thus became evident how much the endless preoccupation with food fills in her emptiness.

Struggling for her independence at the ward, she repeatedly claims: "I don't have enough air." I recall the short breath she suffered as a child and mirror the sense that there is not enough "pure oxygen" outside to keep her alive. She cannot trust that whoever is out there is there for her, able to see her, to sense her and thereby enables her to exist as an individual. On the one hand, she feels that without insisting on her loneliness and strength, she would be lost. On the other hand, when she finally gets a long-aspired vacation, after immense struggles, she is filled with terror of the loneliness and emptiness within. She is anxious about leaving the ward and it turns out that within, too, "there is no oxygen."

Only after months she lets some of her friends visit her and lets herself be empty in their presence, sad and heavy, without faking as she usually does. She also goes out alone at night and lets herself connect with the emptiness she senses without running away. One evening, she dances alone in the dark with a sense of freedom she hadn't remembered. She also took afternoon naps, relaxation she never previously allowed herself, but she still fills herself with preoccupations against the emptiness and fails to gain weight.

In a harsh confrontation, her doctor says angrily that she has wasted our time and the insurer's money, and unless she gains weight, she would have to leave the ward. Sheryl, with new ability to recognize her feelings, felt insulted and belittled. She translates his message like this: "You are here as a charity case, you are dependent on me, and it's on my terms that I'll keep you here or kick you out."

On her parents' visit, she told them that she was determined to work upon discharge in order to avoid taking their money and was hurt by her father's response calling her manipulative. She ran away crying but tried to listen to herself, and then realized that she felt her father belittled the same exact Spartan-like character she worked so hard to establish in order to win his attention. She went back and confronted him with this insight and feeling she was filled with.

Before she left the ward, I suggested that she might consider the idea of using the feeding tube. The tube was attractive because all the years she worked hard to reach the "sublime" status of being severely ill. She surprises herself when she now fights the illness desperately. I mirror that and explain both parts: the archaic longing to be totally dependent and taken care of, while needing the near-death justification for that, and the persistence of keeping control as a means for self-maintenance absent any trust in people. On the one hand, Sheryl is terrified at the prospects of leaving the ward: "I don't have my own self to be with." On the other hand, she cannot trust the staff. Her parents strongly object to her discharge. She is preoccupied with their response and their "grieving looks" but nonetheless chooses to leave. Once she makes her decision, I mirror her authentic choice made from within, despite its pathological elements.

Sheryl moves to Jerusalem. The days of preparations are filled with deep sadness and loneliness. She fills the emptiness by cooking and reading cookbooks and adheres to a strict routine organized around her meals and sessions at Hadassah. Her treatment schedule serves as an excuse not to meet anyone.

She describes her sleeping difficulties and forces herself to go to bed when she is nearly exhausted. I mirror her fear to stop "doing" and to let go, fearing that she would lose the ground of her identity and find herself with an un-held self and existential fear of disappearance. In response, Sheryl relates to the wish for someone to be there, to hold her and to hug her. She increasingly uses the therapeutic relationship as a source for holding: she doesn't miss a moment of the sessions and experiences them as "oxygen." Her terror of leaving the ward is manifested, among other things, in her apparent effort to work hard in the sessions to secure her place with me. The developing transference is "mirror transference," at the very primary level of "merger" (Kohut, 1977b). Sheryl speaks quietly, uses sophisticated metaphors and lowers her eyes. I am attuned and fully committed to the effort of understanding and mirroring from within. The transference is complicated because apparently, she makes no demands and it seems she expects nothing of me. Nonetheless, I am no less cautious than her, unspontaneous, afraid to "miss" and offer inaccurate mirroring. My sense of commitment in light of her severe physical condition, loneliness, anxiety and her hopes from the treatment, leaves no room for other feelings inside me.

Gradually, we come to know her "self-guilt" (Goodsitt, 1997). This feeling has accompanied her since her childhood, telling her that she has no right to take up space. Sheryl recollects childhood memories: a memory she has of being on an eighth-grade field trip – there was not enough room and some of the children were taken off the bus. The entire day she felt a strong feeling of doing something bad, of taking someone else's place. A memory from high school in which she rose from her seat at the family dinner table, and her father looked at her and said "Sheryl, you developed a rear end." In Hebrew, this phrase connotes high hatting, with a sexual innuendo. Sheryl immediately fell deep down into her anorexia, and ever since then, whenever someone refers to her gaining weight, she goes on a hunger strike.

Upon rising up from the table that day, Sheryl read disappointment in her father's look. She felt he wanted her to stay forever slim and graceful – "something angelic, sublime." I translate it to an existence that takes no space, unsexual, never growing and not autonomous.

Sheryl describes her childhood as completely immersed in other people's grief. She used to collect every newspaper article on kidnapped children or fallen soldiers and imagine herself as part of the plot. She saw it as an opportunity to assimilate the grief, which accompanies her "for no reason" – "like I was born grieving." We understand her identification with the dead as being attracted to the aura of those not occupying any space.

Several months later, when she is totally dedicated to a friend suffering from cancer, she raises her fears that her friend would either die or get healthy. In both cases, Sheryl would be left lonely, emptied and insignificant. She can feel that she belongs and exists only as a selfobject for others, that is, she must feel needed to feel any self-worth. She works as a nurse for a physically disabled lady and feels like a servant, but then realizes that she herself initiates humiliating services she was never asked to perform. When her mood gets better, she arrives at the clinic one day feeling elevated by the spring and the holiday, but her good experience is ruined when she sees her "swollen" face in the mirror. Again, I point out the lack of legitimacy to take up space and enjoy herself, while her disappearance, on the other hand, embodied by her anorexia, fulfills the family expectation thus endowing her with a sense of identity.

Her anorexia is her declaration of autonomy.

> It is the only thing in which I do what I want. If I give up on my anorexia, I will be just like everybody else and lose my self. The person I am today is the anorexia. I devoted many years to it, fostered it, worked on it, and without it I will be left with nothing.

Contrary to her principles, and following our talks, Sheryl dares to ask her brother for equipment for her motor scooter. She is insulted by his refusal, and soon her anger and stinging pain make room for feelings of emptiness and pointlessness. She is convinced that she really deserves nothing and then she feels like she has nothing inside her. Her internal presumption is that she is worthless. She is therefore highly attentive and alert to her environment and puts many efforts in feeling worthy. In therapy, at this point, she dares to take a greater risk of getting closer and fully express her emotions, sometimes warmly, although the overall feeling is still somewhat distant.

Alongside the mirror transference, over time it seems that an idealization transference (Kohut, 1977b) gradually emerges to the surface. This transference, too, is highly complicated. Although we are both deeply invested in the therapy and perceive it as important, and although Sheryl sees me as professional and endowing her with confidence, I still feel increasingly helpless about the gap between our conversations and the absence of any actual change in practice. Despite her beautiful insights in therapy, Sheryl gradually and slowly begins to lose weight again.

Sheryl is very concerned about protecting me in therapy so I would continue to believe in her and wouldn't give up on her. When I urge her to share her feelings with me, she feels I am tired of her, that I am losing my patience and sharing my feelings with other team members behind her back. In an attempt to arouse my interest, she talks about her neediness, but she doesn't let herself to genuinely turn me into a selfobject who is responsible and trustworthy, and on whom she can lean on, in order to let anything grow inside her.

During most of the sessions, she looks down. I mirror the longing entailed in her look. Longing for someone powerful, real and trustworthy, someone who is there for her, that she shouldn't take care of him or the situation. Very slowly, she discloses her yearning for serenity, for some rest. To let herself rest within a relationship means to trust, but to rest in general means to be "a parasite." Both states are completely illegitimate. Her attraction to death can now be understood as longing for somewhere to be enveloped by because in the hands of death, one can totally and fully let go.

Sheryl finds it hard to understand her sense of worthlessness and self-guilt, as well as her difficulty to rest, against the backdrop of her childhood. She used to be the "queen" of the house, enjoyed a central place, acted tyrannically and did as she pleased. The explanation she came up with was the gap between her privileged status at home and her encounter with the outside world. In school, she suddenly realized that she was only one among many others. She felt lost, and absent any affirmative looks around her she also felt ugly and disliked. I raise some doubts about her "queenship." What kind of a queen is so attentive to the needs of her "subordinates" and so sensitive to their looks? What kind of a queen has to stomp her feet and struggle so persistently to get what she wants? Sheryl had no figures to count on to meet her needs and set some boundaries. Absent any confidence that such holding would be available, at a very young age she assumed responsibility and control; and absent attentiveness, she became stubborn and demanding. Sheryl defined her monarchy through her deprivations. She discovered that this way she was able to "take up space" in her father's mind, who adored determination and relentlessness. Her monarchy, which started absent an ideal parental image, turned into enslavement to a façade of uniqueness.

Her downward look in our sessions also proves to set her free from the need to maintain her façade, from her dependence on her father's "constitutive look." Following this exploration, Sheryl began, slowly, to take up more space, and separate from her family. Home does not "call" her as before. She still goes there only on the weekends, unwillingly. Her sleeping problems, which have already improved in the city, worsen at home. She keeps herself busy baking until dawn, then works in the farm when she is exhausted. She connects to her family through giving, but then she is "worn out." Home becomes her refuge from the outside world, in which she still fails to fit in. Perceiving her objects as fragile and emptied leaves her guilt-stricken, facing the need to abandon them, and she lacks the resources to establish connections outside her home. However, at the same time she manages to get less involved in the increasing family tensions. She is also less patient toward her father and less preoccupied in the way she is perceived. When I mirror those buds of self, Sheryl talks about her fear that "this bud would bloom" – her fear of developing delight, health, independence, spontaneity because those equal detachment and loneliness.

Her idealizing transference deepens. I feel like I read into her, and one word of mine is sometimes all it takes to enlighten the broader picture for her. She lets herself raise spontaneous, unorganized thoughts, and it does not bother her as much as before. Her looks and smile are more open. Her affect is fuller, and her voice sometimes breaks down and tears come up. She feels that our sessions are the only occasions in which she totally lets herself be herself.

After five months of living in the city, Sheryl starts to meet people. She concludes that this is her way out of the illness. She goes on a blind date for the first time in her life. Her "angelic-morbid" distinctive appearance becomes ego-dystonic (alienated from the ego). Sheryl dares more to ask for an explicit feedback rather than scan her surroundings like a radar and stay confused, and overall, she feels like "she begins to live." With her parents, however, she keeps the old status quo. With them, she still needs the illness to allow herself to rest instead of doing any required activity, such as rubbing her father's aching back.

At this point, she starts to lose weight rather quickly and feels weak. She is more aware of her alarming physical condition. Physical anxieties emerge, fearing a heart failure and collapsing in the street. She suddenly feels vulnerable riding her small motor scooter in busy roads. Her feelings of omnipotence and indifference about her body are replaced with powerful anxiety, but it does not lead to any practical change. On the contrary, she undertakes additional jobs and does not increase her food intake accordingly.

In this phase of therapy, I invest my soul but face a stone wall. Beyond the façade of impressive therapeutic work and close relationship, death is still in the air. I find myself extremely cautious, suffocating my spontaneity, totally attuned to her and nonetheless wherever I turn I face a sense of dead end and guilt. When I am swept away with the façade, I am practically neglecting Sheryl, and when her condition deteriorates, I feel guilty for not really seeing her and not setting boundaries, just like her mother. When I have a complaint about her, I too, like her mother, can never be satisfied despite her efforts. Alternatively, when she asks to continue and see me in my private clinic after I terminate my work at the outpatient clinic, and I pose some conditions and demand she reaches 40 kg – again I am loaded with guilt because I impose my will threatening to leave her, just like her father.

Supervision is extremely helpful for me in my efforts to return my self to myself, to take up space, to let myself feel my anger at her and believe in my right to establish some boundaries in order to protect her. All this even at the price of discomfort, disappointment and break of our "idyllic" relationship.

When I increasingly share these emotional processes with Sheryl, a surge of new vitality enters our relationship. It allows memories to emerge, and feelings toward her parents that were more distant from consciousness can now be acknowledged, put into words and given room. For the first time, Sheryl relates a memory of a nightmare, in which she wakes up with a round face, but her family treats her like a healthy person and cease to attend to her. Her feeling toward therapy in this dream is that the professional team lost control over her weight and her body is increasingly swelling, although she accurately followed the plan. In the transference, Sheryl reenacts her experience of the seducing, promising home that turns out to be empty. I mirror her fury: "The food you give me here is only seemingly nutritious, only seemingly fulfilling, but in fact it only swells me, it is nothing but air, all of it."

At this point, I want to work on her miserliness. Sheryl is not able to spend a penny on others and barely on herself. She lives in a sense of siege and the need to reserve for emergency. She gives her parents a shopping list and takes all she needs from them. Along with her guilt feelings, she also feels her internal demand for compensation and revenge. Not gaining weight is also understood as part of this "not giving." Sheryl is a prisoner of deprivation, directs her anger at herself and indirectly conveying the message to those around her: "You'd be dead sorry for my death." Her fury is elusive and terrifying. She touches it and then withdraws: "I have anger at the foundation of everything. The foundation is rotten, and I try to grow beautiful things on it." Immediately after that, she says: "But how can I be angry at them? This isn't fair, they gave us the best they knew." She indirectly expresses her anger and simultaneously dismisses it. By taking anything from her parents, she also accepts their tight grip. When she asks me to complement 15 minutes of a session she had to cut shorter because "any minute here is precious for me" – the compliment nearly hides her aggression. In any event, she is tormented by guilt. She is so preoccupied with the fear that I'd leave her that she cannot connect to her anger at me. Beyond anger she is filled with terror to be left alone, in front of an indifferent audience, even indifferent to her anger. This fear fosters the anger and neutralizes it at once.

Transforming from merger with me to a bigger separation from me as a selfobject (Kohut, 1977b), I am not as comforting as before and further emphasizing the conflict. At present, I don't only empathically mirror her feeling of abuse, a feeling that negated her ability to give, but also challenge her to give, including gaining weight, not out of self-deprecation but as a form of taking up space; not as a pleasing selfobject but to free herself from the chains of her deprivation and anger.

A month is left until the termination of therapy within the outpatient clinic and the move to my private clinic. Several months earlier, we agreed that she must reach a minimum weight, which is not life-threatening, in order to move to a private setting because I cannot assume responsibility for a patient in such a poor physical condition. At this stage, the feasibility of her meeting this condition and reaching 40 kg in a month is unrealistic. Sheryl firmly refuses to hospitalize herself, and it is clear that forced hospitalization would not be effective in her case. I agree to compromise and to see her for an additional month in the outpatient clinic, although I no longer work there. We sign a contract that Sheryl drafts herself, stipulating that she must gain 2.5 kg over the next eight weeks to continue in a private setting.

After several sessions in which she expressed her difficulty "to give" and understanding it together in the light of the feeling of being used and extorted all her life, with the only form of giving she knows is as a selfobject, she tells me for the first time, with great shame and pain, about her tendency "to take." In her past, there was an episode in which she was caught by a surveillance camera while stealing "diet" products from a supermarket. Today, in her workplace, she often "sneaks" little things into her bag. The question "will I be caught? Will they discover who I really am beyond the façade of the dedicated worker?" is challenging, and this challenge gives her a sense of vitality, along with a heavy burden of guilt, shame and fear.

Sheryl raises her concern that by revealing this secret to me, I would be afraid that she'd take from me as well. I say that she is checking, here with me, how long would the "façade of the dedicated therapist" hold on, when the revenge and compensation wishes dwell inside; the wish to take and take more and more and never give anything. The shift to private therapy, which she would have to finance by herself, also marks a shift to a more mutual negotiation of giving between the two of us, which still infuriates her.

Being a selfless selfobject, Sheryl does not only feel the necessity to give, but is also deprived of the "freedom to receive." She can either receive or take only through hidden extortion, thefts, or loss of control entailed in bulimia, rather than in a healthy, joyful and guiltless manner.

A hidden sense of entitlement is active beyond the conscious feeling of disentitlement. I feel it increasingly in the sessions. Sheryl asks for special requests, always past the session's 50 minutes. For example, she asks me to continue to see her at the clinic if she receives the insurer's approval, or that I would arrange for a meeting with a nurse even though she cannot pay for it. I feel very committed to accept these requests because they are presented gently, with the confidence that she would be rejected. I feel increasingly pressured, but at this point I do not offer any interpretation.

Sheryl brings new tones, which I try to echo strongly. Her manager asked her to replace her heavy shoes with more feminine shoes. She spontaneously resisted, protested and demanded that he'd pay for these shoes if they mattered to him. In the past, she would obey, secretly infuriated inside, and seek revenge behind his back with petty thefts, or alternatively she would refuse and resign.

During this period, she also tells me, again with embarrassment and shame, that she showed off her new haircut to her manager. I positively mirror the feminine vitality she allowed herself to express and her ability to choose to be a woman by her own determination and to choose otherwise when she doesn't feel like it – just like in the shoes incident.

A month before we ended the therapy at the outpatient clinic, at the beginning of one session, Sheryl examines the way I look at her – to check whether she seems to me happy or tired – and reports that she lost 0.5 kg and that her current weight is 37 kg. She begs in tears that I continue to believe in her. She fears the end of treatment and is preoccupied with the question whether I gave up on her. The mystery of losing weight is now the focus of the sessions.

Again, Sheryl talks much about her compulsive visits at her parents' house over the weekends, and about her need of her mother's gaze. "Just like that, without it, I don't know how I . . . look . . . behave." She examines whether she looks to her mother tired or happy, words that sound very familiar to me. At the same moment, she recalls a frequent childhood fantasy – that her parents are dead. She often played with this thought as a child and felt guilty for the sense of relief it invoked.

I ask her what she would feel if she gained weight as planned and Sheryl replies: "If I gain weight now it will be your success. . . . It's weird, it's something that I, too, want badly. . . . But if I get better there, the gratification will be yours, not mine." I interpreted her distrust that if she does anything that I also look forward to – she would still be able to stay herself. The relief invoked by the childhood fantasy is now well-understood: "You feel that only if they are dead you will start living. Maybe here as well you need me to 'die' – be out of your life – so it can be your life." The thought about getting better outside therapy does bring some immediate relief, but soon she also talks about the "bubble" she might get back to and acknowledges the heavy toll of isolation and detachment she feels she must have to feel she has a selfhood. The selective approvals she received from her parents – within the limit of their own needs – left her feeling that anything she does satisfies others. As a chronic selfobject, she is afraid that gaining weight now will also be to please me.

In the remaining four weeks, we work intensively on maternal transference. At this stage, we understand that just as her father wanted to see her as an ideal reflection of himself – by turning her to strong and stubborn – her mother, coming from a grieving family and attempting to deny her own depression – wanted a cheerful, lively daughter. In her sickness and sadness, Sheryl expresses her fury and resistance to her mother. "I don't want her to be delighted, I don't want to please her." This way she maintains her selfhood.

But soon it turns out that things are more complicated. Unlike her father, whose pride in his eyes was evident when Sheryl met his expectations, her mother's look was frozen and reflected nothing when Sheryl was lively and independent. In Sheryl's words, her mother encouraged her to go out and enjoy herself, but when Sheryl obeyed, her mother emotionally withdrew and forgot her. Sheryl transfers to me her feeling that if she recovers, I would be pleased and fail to keep in mind that she has other distresses, too. Not only would she lose herself while pleasing me, but she would be deleted and emptied facing my failure to see her. On the other hand, as a sick person she would present me with a "professional challenge" and this is the only way she can maintain my interest in her. Through the transference, we are introduced to another layer of her mother, probably a lot less conscious, in which Sheryl was an object for projection of morbid parts of sadness, emptiness and death. These parts, embodied through Sheryl's sickness and pain, invoked a stronger response from her mother, who reacted with concern and empathy. More than anything, it was this response that gave Sheryl a sense of existence and distinctive identity. Her big sad eyes had a reputation in the family and earned her a sense of uniqueness. Only when she touches death, she wins a sense of life. Her sickness, just like the risk of getting caught stealing, gave her a sense of vitality and selfhood through resisting the overt expectations from her. The trap was that this behavior matched her mother's less overt expectations, thus rewarded her with attention and a sense of existence, but again she lost her selfhood.

Sheryl finds herself in a similar catch-22 in therapy as well. She feels that if she gains weight, she would please me. It will be my professional success, and thereby she would lose her selfhood and be forgotten by me. Staying sick was apparently her only way to maintain her selfhood, but this would also please me, satisfy my interest and challenge, and she believes that this is the only way for her to earn room in my heart.

I mirror the catch-22 in which she always lives through others, sick or healthy, sad or happy, and now I challenge her to pick a third option – live through her self, believe in the selfhood inside her and make her choices out of this selfhood, rather than through obedience or resistance to someone outside her. This option entails great pain of giving up her wish that her parents would be involved in her growth.

Sheryl finds it extremely hard to let go of her wish to be filled by her home. She is drawn to her home like a black hole, a draw that relates to her will to repair the most significant relationships of her life, and through them – repair herself. "I need my home, as if I haven't fully exhausted what's in there, what could have been there. I must breathe the house as much as I can." This draw is also related to an unequivocal message she received from her mother, which she shares with me for the first time: "You have only one home." She fears that if she separates herself from her home, including the feelings of emptiness and failure it entails, she will find nothing outside, and home itself will also fall apart.

I feel that she tries to hold on to me in the same provocative way through not gaining weight; through the void, the emptiness and the refusal to give. I prefer, at this stage, to offer an experience-near interpretation: "How painful would it be to feel the grief for what you never got and would never get from home, and how painful would it be to leave your parents alone with this emptiness."

My call for her recovery immediately relates to leaving her alone to return to the race of life, requiring total and superhuman strength. The disabilities connected with her sickness protected her from that. With no physical justification, it is clear to her that she wouldn't allow herself to continue her therapy. I point out the double fear of physical recovery, on the one hand because of her distrust that I will still be interested in her and attentive to her, including her difficulties and distresses, and on the other hand because of her assumption that as a healthy person she would have to switch immediately to her father's strict standards, leave therapy and deny any need of hers.

This is the first time it occurs to her that I sincerely wait for her to be physically healthy. She recalls how she once read in the look of her

acupuncturist the facial expression of her mother each time she entered
the room. It was clear to her that unless her physical condition is ter-
rible, she would have no right to lie on the bed and receive therapy.
This feeling was repeated, in several versions, in all kinds of treatments.
She is emotionally touched and saying: "Suddenly it is clear to me that
I want therapy that wouldn't focus on life and death. I want a therapy
of life, of quality of life." In fact, she keeps saying that within a human
relationship all she knows is a selfless existence; existence of an abyss,
of sickness, of siege, and this is the only way she is able to exist within
therapy.

Sheryl suddenly realizes that through her dead end, she avoids confronting the familiar past experiences – her fear of not being able to stop
eating once she started; her hatred toward her body; the distressing preoccupation in thoughts about food; and mainly, the need to cope with
the looks of others. Sheryl says:

> I went through major changes. I am not as empty as I was, but I'm
> not sure that the self I have is enough. I am afraid that the candle is
> still tiny and wouldn't be enough to light my way.

I answered:

> I feel that the internal change you underwent can already enable
> you to cope through patterns less destructive than before. I can
> believe in you, the self within you, which is growing stronger and
> is able today to cope in a healthier manner, but I can't believe in you
> instead of you, and I can't choose instead of you to bear the pains
> change entails.

In the last session before we terminate, I bring up forcefully the center
of her pathology – the self-guilt that emerges any time she lets go of the
selfless selfobject position – and acknowledges her self.

> My parents are so helpless and suffering – being used by my sib-
> lings, don't know how to set boundaries, how can I watch them like
> that, and get away from them instead of protecting them? It is unfair
> that I live my life and they will be left so helpless.

And I reply:

> You feel that if you leave your parents their ship will drown, and you
> are willing to drown with them. You can't believe they can cope on

their own, and if you are not living their life you feel tremendous guilt. I also see you suffering, needy, quite helpless in the face of your illness, can't set your own boundaries, but I can't live your life instead of you, or keep you alive instead of you, regardless of how badly I want to. Furthermore, I believe you can do it on your own, and I'll be happy to walk down this road with you if you let me.

Sheryl left with a strong feeling that she would do anything to return to therapy as soon as possible, along with a feeling that this break is necessary for her own good and there was no other way but confronting all the feelings associated with gaining weight.

Gaining weight is now the main point of gravity in Sheryl's choice to live her life through her self rather than through the pleasing or displeasing of others. The self-guilt on the one hand, and the fury, reckoning and demand to get what was deprived of her, on the other hand, are powerful forces that Sheryl's growing self must now face.

7   The Therapist's Position Facing a Grandiose Self

Michal Man

In this chapter, I would like to discuss a therapeutic issue that I encountered while treating a patient with severe narcissistic disorder. The patient sought therapy for her bulimia nervosa, purging type, and the issue that was raised concerned the therapeutic handling of a grandiose-exhibitionist self with grotesque manifestations.

Tara (the patient changed her given name) is a 37-year-old divorced woman, suffering from bulimia since her early adolescence, with varying severity of her symptoms. She works in the field of sports and martial arts, she is very slim looking and dresses and moves provocatively.

At the beginning of therapy, with a long history of failed and fragmented therapeutic attempts, Tara showed considerable resistance to providing background details during the intake interview. "I raised myself, I was born from earth, family doesn't exist in my case." She started sharing a little more information about her family only after nine months of therapy.

Tara was one of the youngest children in a big family of a Kurdish descent. Her childhood memories revolve around feelings of loneliness, inferiority and deprivation. "I couldn't find anything special about myself, I wasn't the most beautiful, neither the oldest nor the youngest."

She grew up in the shadow of a father casting terror on the family. Her father is an alcoholic and violent, and his figure is encompassed by shame. Tara is ambivalent toward him. She strongly identifies with some of the traits attributed to him, such as manipulation, evilness, jealousy and loneliness, along with a partially conscious dream to please him and thereby to change him. This dream is related to a family myth told by Tara's mother, according to which the father started to cheat on the mother upon Tara's birth. This myth resonates with the supernatural powers Tara attributes to herself. Sometimes these powers are demonic: she "casts an evil eye," and sometimes these are supernatural healing abilities: "I bring the best out of people."

Tara is preoccupied with the question whether her father sees her as a saint or as a prostitute. This question haunts her in her ample, intense and unstable relationships with men. These relationships are characterized by vigorous and seductive courtship on her part, trying to turn men who are self-absorbed and who are using her into devoted and caring partners. This attitude was accompanied by a sense of self-humiliation denied by self-grandiosity along with severe devaluation of those men.

Tara is also confused and ambivalent toward her mother. Her story relates a highly narcissistic and manipulative mother figure, who indeed took care of her children physically, particularly around food, but was emotionally detached. Tara's mother used to degrade Tara's father, overshadow him and actively arouse his jealousy. Both parents failed to provide clear intergenerational boundaries. Tara switched between them with alternate feelings of empathy, pity, concern and admiration for one of them while respectively demonizing the other, and vice versa.

As a child, Tara was quiet and observant. At home, she witnessed shouts, quarrels and violence around her, and in school, she would stare with wide thirsty eyes at her "rich, clean, beautiful and smart" classmates. In school, she was obedient and barely spoke out loud, and at home, she made up for it by chattering endlessly and by gathering her siblings around her to hear her stories and fantasies. Over the years, Tara has put immense energies into establishing a façade of uniqueness, which entailed lies and various attempts to impress.

In her adolescence, Tara was sent to a *kibbutz*, a communitarian-agricultural village in Israel, where she resided and studied with the local youth. Again, she experienced unbearable feelings of envy and inferiority. She took gym classes where she stood out for her talents and she started to dedicate herself to them. She spent many hours practicing, always taking some fans with her as an audience. She totally devoted herself to working on her fitness and athletic skills, participated in national competitions and won great success. At the same time, she developed an eating disorder, which started as anorexia and soon turned into bulimia. Her investment in her body was immense: its appearance, its weight, what goes in and out, its athletic abilities and its seduction capability.

Tara studied physical education and currently works in this field. Her first days in new educational and work environments are typically characterized by making huge impression, which soon shatters down and leaves her feeling rejected and reacting with typical grandiosity and far-reaching devaluations.

When starting her therapy, Tara suffered severe symptoms of bingeing and vomiting, whose frequency was absolutely dependent on her relations with rapidly alternating men. She was also addicted to impulsive and promiscuous sexual behavior. Similar to her use of food, Tara used men for self-regulation and for filling her inner emptiness, and they, in turn, used her for their needs.

I got the impression of a woman feeling lost and lonely, a woman whose internal regulation mechanisms are fundamentally flawed and who needs immediate and concrete satisfaction. She talked in an enthusiastic, dramatic and overwhelming manner, quite associative, often pseudo-philosophical, loud and vibrant, while totally immersed in her efforts to define herself and impress me.

In most sessions, she was in a near-hypomanic state, with euphoric feelings of power, energy and optimism. She perceived herself as an artist and looked glorious. Alternatively, there were few sessions in which she looked pale and dimmed and brought feelings of total defeat in all arenas, emptiness and collapse of her self-worth, amounting to despair and suicidal feelings. But in most cases, her threat of feeling depressed was so strong that she filled the sessions with cheerful content, without any room to crack her defenses.

Her main preoccupation was with her self-worth and gaining the acknowledgment of others. Likewise, a considerable confusion of her experiences was apparent, and there were rapid and dramatic changes in her attitude toward people around her, toward her goals and toward her ideals. She was enslaved by a fantasy of a Prince Charming who would lift her from rock bottom, discover what a noble princess she is and finally shower her with the treatment she deserves, which she had never received.

Tara was ambivalent toward the men who were attracted to her, who disclosed their feelings and vulnerability and who adored her. On the other hand, she idealized those relationships where she was attracted to men who were indifferent and abusive. Quite often, she found their looks to resemble her father's and unconsciously talked about them with the same terminology that she used to describe her father: "I want to prove to him that I am no whore," "I want to make him realize who Tara is." She was playing with fantasies of compensating for his faults and making him appreciate her.

The narcissistic transference was in the most primitive level of merger with an ideal and omnipotent selfobject. Tara shared in great detail what she experienced in between sessions, while giving defensive-grandiose and devaluative interpretations to the incidents she encountered. In the countertransference, I often felt lonely, unnecessary in the room and abused. Throughout these sessions, I occasionally felt myself fading in the presence of self-absorbed Tara, and at the end of such sessions, I felt overwhelmed and at the same time completely emptied.

Tara was totally and immensely demanding toward me yet conveyed that she does not need anything from me. She denied any need of others. She repeated many times, within her grandiose trance, that she was the one to do all the work in therapy by herself; she ignored transference-oriented interpretations, interrupted me and seemed inattentive. The only sign of noticing my interventions was the associative increase of her grandiosity as a reaction to an insignificant detail of what I said that was experienced as harming her self-image.

Many times, I felt that my words were disturbing her, emphasizing the distance between us and the otherness, whereas what she actually needed was full merger and partnership with a sense of security. Despite the great chaos characterizing Tara's sessions and her life, she showed up regularly every week.

The therapeutic metaphor that helped me to maintain my therapeutic and interpretative position rather than fade away in her presence was the model of children's play therapy. Tara was like a child playing on her own and ignoring the adult's presence, but the interpretations given by that adult are effectively received. Only on rare occasions, mainly when she was in touch with the inferior stance in the vertical split (Kohut, 1977b), she would stare at me with her big eyes and thirstily absorb my empathic mirroring and the links I made to her past. But also in the other kind of sessions, which were the majority, in which she was on a self "trip," mirroring was offered. The mirroring mainly reflected the fact that her source of vigor and liveliness was external.

At the time, Tara totally rejected my attempts to touch the painful side of the split and to connect her to her depressed self that showed up in times where there was no one to please her with his love.

The sessions were always too short for her and she unconsciously tried to ignore the clock and extend the session. She tried to take additional things as well, other than my time. She often asked to make a phone call from my room or asked for a cup of coffee, which immediately aroused feelings of aggression and rejection toward her. Her self-absorption, demandingness and abusiveness disgusted me. In my heart, I blamed her of any good thing being ruined around her, and I empathized with the people who pushed her away.

To resume my therapeutic stance, I repeatedly envisioned baby Tara, who couldn't find her own face in the face of her mother. Or toddler Tara who couldn't find gleam in the eyes of those surrounding her, who rejects anyone and misses family dinners just to be noticed, to no avail. Only this way could I interpret her requests from me in the spirit of: "You feel that you still want to be in the phase of receiving," or "You lack so much that you must keep on taking." Only after I envisioned girl Tara could I offer such interpretations out of a genuine empathy and understanding that she truly cannot do anything but receive. Even when she said over and over again that she did all the therapeutic work by herself, I warmly interpreted that she was so used to being in a position of not getting anything and that she must act for herself.

Over time, Tara expressed her discontent of certain abusive and manipulative behaviors of hers. She was also more attentive to social feedback she received for her excessive flow of speech. In a group floor exercise at her gym class, she found herself "at the center but alone" and asked to learn how to connect with people. She began to bring to the sessions more and more confrontations she had with people over her self-absorption and her inability to give. Mostly she avoided confronting those contents in the session by shifting into grandiose associations, through a vortex of confusion and contradictions: "I am simple," "I don't even need relationships," "I am too complex for relationships," "I connect with anyone, from the poorest worker to the brightest professor." In those moments, when I manage to get out of the tide surrounding me, I persist with interpretations in the spirit of: "You talk so much about yourself and compliment yourself because it is hard for you to believe that someone out there will be attuned to you and compliment you."

Among other self-doubts and reflections, Tara was preoccupied with the question of her sanity, for behaviors like her intensive courtship of a famous actor who took advantage of her and used her; or hanging out with three men in one night. I want to comfort her by saying "I don't think you are crazy, but it's difficult for you to be, and to stay, with hard feelings. You have to do very dramatic things just to avoid these feelings," but Tara does not allow us the space to discuss it. Immediately, in an increasing flood, she replies to herself: "This is me, I am special." "I am more normal than most people I know and most psychologists, I teach the psychologists, I also taught you a lot." When I manage to overcome my aversion and revenge feelings, to calm myself down and not without effort to put my self psychology glasses back on, I can comfort her as I planned.

Feeling superior, Tara experiences all others as being nurtured by her. Like a classic narcissistic mother, who is also gratified by the baby she nurtures, like me in therapy listening and mirroring – she enjoyed showering her influence. However, when she did not get anything in return, she experienced others as parasites sucking her up and emptying her and she reacted in an uncontrolled fury.

After several months in therapy, better impulse control was emerging, and she showed a slightly improved ability for introspection. In the sessions, she still tries to "steal" minutes, admirations etc. in a coercive manner, and I often feel abused and humiliated, but sometimes she also expresses her wishes, for instance for a cup of coffee, while saying that she avoids asking. She also talks about situations of feeling abusive and almost like a thief.

Later on, Tara talks about a sense of moderation in her life. She listens to others much more and feels capable for such giving because she knows I always listen to her. "You are the only person with whom I really talk about myself." I hope that she will indeed increasingly channel her admiration needs into our relationship rather than throw them at any one around. But soon my hopes are frustrated when Tara enters an extremely chaotic period. Every week she comes up with a story about a new guy, to whom her mystic powers led her. She fits herself to him like a chameleon. With one guy she becomes religious, to another she gives oral sex and is drawn to an orgy with him, with a third she becomes an orthodox vegan and the next day, with the fourth, she practices shooting for hunting purposes. These short affairs all end exactly the same; they end when the guy doesn't call her or otherwise harms her and she devaluates him and anything related to him.

Simultaneously, Tara is looking for a job in her profession and is repeatedly rejected, or, if admitted, is soon fired. Unable to bear this stinging pain, her binges and purges worsen and she feels like a "wide open hole." In our sessions, she becomes particularly theatrical, boasting to me with her talents and performance. Her striking surprise – how is it possible that people were not impressed by her or realized her value – is rather pathetic. If it wasn't for going over my notes where I cited her, I would find it hard to believe I indeed heard such sentences. Among other things, she said, "it was genius what I told him, brilliant, and this idiot didn't even understand," or "I am so talented, genius, even before I read Nietzsche and Jung I said exactly what they said. I even wrote down some of the stuff. Only that when they said it – they won global praise, and when I said it – no one paid attention." In the sessions, Tara continues to think that she is constantly rediscovering herself, her eyes are shining and she is totally in love with herself. Any gentle push to a more introspective position is rejected within her incessant talking.

In supervision, I yell "help me, I'm drowning!" I say that I can't connect with her or find any thread that would help me connect to her, and I feel very worried. My instinct tells me to burst her bubble. This increasing need of mine is also a revenge for her using me for her needs without seeing me at all. Supervision helps me to keep in mind that if

I confront her with reality, I will reenact her early trauma, when her parents failed to confirm her grandiosity. Thanks to that I manage, from time to time, to be empathic to her pain for not being echoed. Instead of bursting her grandiosity, I mirror: "How painful it is when others fail to acknowledge your talent" or "How hurtful it is that he can't see your beautiful parts." To a large extent, I thus join forces with Tara's flawed judgment, but despite the unease of this position, I keep on standing by the self rather than by the ego. In this period, I often ask myself if anything of what I say gets to her at all, since Tara keeps on ignoring my words as she talks enthusiastically.

Whenever Tara starts a new relationship, which happens at least once a week, she shifts between immense fear of abandonment, resulting in a binge, and denial of the difficulty and a pseudo-philosophical defense, according to which "the most important thing is the present moment, it doesn't matter if anything comes out of it, and in any event I don't even know if I look for an exclusive relationship." A minute later, she insists that if she has one steady relationship she won't vomit, and I agree with her that food answers a deep hunger, far beyond physical hunger. She once said, without sensing the symbolic quality of her words, "when the house is full – I won't eat much, and if it's empty – I will empty it altogether."

One day Tara calls me, asking to extend the length of our session. I agree, and in the session, I interpret that she needed to receive a lot, more than usual, but this time she chose to satisfy this hunger through our relationship, a human connection, rather than through food – which is a breakthrough.

She often asks me for approvals for her actions and her self-definition: "What do you think about the message I left him?" "Do you think I am an artist?" She also starts a journal, as a potential substitution for binges, which she is convinced would soon become a world best seller.

Her improving condition and her progress in therapy are very delusive. A good period is soon accompanied by a period of total confusion about her achievements and relationships. She phones the clinic urgently, demands to call me and is furious when I am not immediately available. Her voice becomes cold and demanding and she often makes suicidal insinuations to engage me. In her relationships outside the room, she continues to use others as her extensions and is devastated when she is rejected. In therapy, too, I have a constant feeling that she uses me as a container, as a provider of admiration and as an emotional regulation mechanism, but not as her partner in the process of understanding herself. There is no sense of "we" in the therapeutic work.

In one of the sessions, during an attempt on my part to understand her transference, Tara says.

> I feel safe with you, I am comfortable, but this is not an ordinary therapeutic relationship because I use you as a medium. Like a TV transmitter that helps me . . . for this reason I am not going to get angry at you, because this is not an ordinary therapy.

In another session, she says: "Sit down and admire me. I am here not like in the presence of a therapist but like in the presence of a journal to write in." These expressions reflected her need to see me as a selfobject rather than as a separate, independent, object, with a distinct subjectivity. In yet another session, on a rare moment in which she connects to herself, she says:

> I was born an empty vessel, that's why I try to fill myself up with gymnastics. . . . I have to make something of the void, but whatever I do, the vessel is empty and guys sense it and leave me.

Next, Tara starts a relationship with a man whom she decides to marry within a week, in a hurry, fearing that the good might run away. I share her excitement but also try to tone down her impulsivity.

Tara's need of twinship with me is growing. She reads to me letters she received from the man and shows me gifts he gave her. In one session, she suggests that she joins the clinic as a colleague in the field of nutrition and fitness. She feels herself to be an expert, who can contribute to patients with eating disorders no less than their psychotherapists. She wasn't able to become curious about her wish. She was stuck in the fear of rejection and conveys disappointment that hides her anger: "Look, I am not in therapy here. This is studying, I do my work on myself, I have no problem becoming a therapist here." At first, I express my interest in her as a potential colleague for fitness. I ask questions regarding her expertise, what may be her contribution, etc., before I dismiss her suggestion. Collaborating with her pathology, while acknowledging her need of twinship, is effective. Tara never repeats this wish. She only needed the consideration that she can be of use, as equal among equals. To my surprise, at the end of this potentially volatile session, she thanked me warmly, saying, "I learned a lot today."

Tara continues to flood the room with her talk, but the content is less grandiose and it is less rarely that silence is cast upon the room for a few moments, silence that makes room for being. Tara's binges considerably decrease.

Therapy is boosted by Tara's new boyfriend, who is sick of façades, rejects shallow talk, doesn't admire her slimness, her accessories and her dramatic reflections too much, but nonetheless loves her. This is a new and often hard experience for Tara, but she manages to use therapy to observe his attitude from a different perspective. Instead of feeling insulted, she is able to see that he wants her for who she is, rather than for her slim body or athletic talents. Believing that someone is actually interested in her true self was also a terrifying experience. Tara is searching for her identity and frightened that if she gives up her masks, it would turn out to be a void behind them.

In the next couple of months, Tara is involved in finding out what is true and what is false in her life, how much she can regulate herself and to what extent she depends on external regulators. She is much more contained within the new relationship with her boyfriend. In our sessions, she is more present and can have a dialogue with me. She is still drawn often to her narcissistic bubble and makes long enthusiastic speeches about herself, but it is easier to interrupt her and the content is less grandiose. Her behavior also became less impulsive.

Quite soon, however, her boyfriend started to have doubts. He confronted Tara with her problematic sides and with the gap between her outside appearance of a gentle and noble woman, and her behavior at home. Since he delivered his comments without rejecting or scorning her, she was able, to some extent, to discuss them without resorting to massive defenses as she did in the past.

Tara was preoccupied not only by her fear of abandonment but also by her fear of being swallowed up in the relationship. She felt that her merits and strengths inspire her boyfriend, who greatly developed in his profession at this period of time, while she was left without any energy or vibrancy and felt used. Again she fantasizes about Prince Charming, and she longs for the times when she felt anything intensely: delight when she appeared before an audience or painful depression when a boyfriend left her. Now she feels great fear of losing her identity, as diffused and false as it is, and of losing her desire for action. Giving up her old techniques for self-filling leaves her empty and shallow.

Tara then experienced a phase of depression and soul searching. She starts bingeing again and also starts to drink, while fearing she might resemble her alcoholic father. At the same time, driven by the fear that her boyfriend would leave her, she makes dramatic changes in her appearance and gives up her role as the life of the party. The long working through of choosing her body as her ideal representative on earth eventually bears fruit, as she allows herself to gain some weight and quit her obsessive fitness exercises. At this point, she is connected to the worthless, needing, pole, but not as a total downfall. The behavioral changes she made are not apparent yet, but her increasing ability of introspection and willingness to examine her reactions and tone them down, are definitely evident. Tara still expresses her doubts about her boyfriend to anyone who is willing to listen, or brags about a new job before she is even admitted, but she brings these facts to therapy as an object of inquiry. There are touching moments over these months, in which I feel close to her, as she is undergoing a process of separation from her imagined perfectness.

Tara's treatment was terminated after two years because of administrative reasons. The treatment helped in considerably mitigating her eating disorder symptoms. In the last months of therapy, the symptoms could disappear for many weeks and return only upon distress and in a less severe manner. Her grandiosity also toned down to some extent, although it pops up as an available defense when she needs it.

Toward the termination of therapy, the binges drastically worsened and grandiosity showed up again. Tara could not understand how I can give up a remarkable patient like her. She declared her lack of dependence on me and the therapy and used ample manipulations in the last sessions trying to earn more and more sessions, but rejected my proposal to add sessions for which she would pay herself, in addition to the sessions subsidized by the insurance company.

Tara's therapy was characterized by amazing demonstrations of an archaic-grandiose self, like a child who knows nothing but herself. The question was if and how I can be with Tara, to be empathic toward what appeared as a grotesque caricature of shallow grandiosity. The initial impulse was to burst this bubble. My incessant thought was that if it wasn't reality, and the person sitting in front of me did not genuinely and totally believe in the exhibitionist role she performed, it was a rather impressive theater.

The main theoretical issue raised by Tara's treatment was whether to confront her with reality trying to strengthen her ego functions or stay "experience-near" with her. The second option was complicated for the therapist, as it implicated joining forces with an objectively false and quite pathological perspective.

Two difficulties made things all the more complicated. The first was the merger transference, the most primitive mirroring transference referred to by Kohut (1977b). Tara saw me as an unseparated part of herself and left no space between us. I, as a therapist who was completely erased during the sessions, felt greatly tempted to insist on reality check. On the other hand, I needed to fulfill for her the immense, archaic need of a selfobject, totally and for a long time, with no room for myself and respect for my autonomy as a distinct person; and from this position also to foster empathy for her grandiose self. This was a first-rate therapeutic challenge.

The second hurdle was that Tara assigned her selfobject the position of a bystander. She did not wait for any comments but demanded a silent observation of her self-admiration, admiration that many times amounted to a trance of self-enthusiasm.

This manifestation of a self-provider did her a disservice, since it discouraged anyone who had any admiration for her. This left her pumping herself up in a seemingly endless loneliness.

I realized the intensity of my anger and of my feeling of being abused following a dream I had toward the end of Tara's treatment. In my dream, she was walking with two other women and with me. One of the women was holding a bag of fruit and Tara asks her for a pear. Then she asks for another fruit, then another. Before she departed from the three of us, she asks for the fourth fruit, and then I say to her reproachfully: "Why don't you buy yourself a bag of fruit?"

Aside from the dream being my internal summary – how many fruits this therapy yielded and failed to yield – it summarized how difficult it is for a tree that was never nurtured or fostered as a young plant, to yield fruit by itself rather than gather them by demand, and how hard it is to confront this intense demand, the result of such fundamental narcissistic deprivations.

It is clear to me that were the treatment to continue, I would have to invest much effort working through the countertransference, regarding my place as a human being in this treatment.

8 "Living My Life"

Asher Epstein and Dina Roth

Guy was 14 years old when he was referred to us with his parents because of his refusal to eat, suicidal threats and loss of 20 percent of his body weight in the previous year. He was very depressed, saying that there was no point in his life and that only his thinness meant anything. He was diagnosed with anorexia nervosa, restrictive type.

Guy's family consisted of his parents, a younger brother (12 years old) and two little sisters (eight, six). The family immigrated to Israel from France when Guy was six years old. His father, an accountant, suffered financial troubles since the immigration. The mother, a qualified nurse, was working part time. The family resided in an agricultural village in the North of Israel. Because of Guy's refusal to eat at home, his suicidal statements and his depression, he was admitted in the hospital. He was treated with tube-feeding and anti-depressants.

The first phase of his hospitalization witnessed constant attempts to rip the tube off, to leave the ward without permission (in order to jog) and to vomit, along with constant threats of suicide, particularly if he gains weight. To enable Guy's treatment in the open ward, his parents were asked to arrange for a family member to be present all day long.

Guy described himself as suffering inside and said, "even when I'm smiling, a smile is actually not a smile." He expressed his wish to stay little and never grow up and stated that he didn't know who he was. He gave the feeding tube a nickname, thereby expressing his experience that the tube represented his identity.

Guy never acknowledged his right to feel, let alone the possibility of talking about his feelings and expecting someone to listen to them and make room for them. The first task of the therapeutic work was therefore to bring him to the point where he can acknowledge his right to feel, and let himself articulate his feelings and wishes, without having to search for other, destructive, ways to express them.

Guy's treatment included individual therapy, family therapy, group therapy and parent counseling. The entire therapeutic framework shared the same objective: to give Guy the space to acknowledge that he is a human being with needs, wishes and emotions and help him believe in his right to be himself and to develop so as to realize his own identity. Guy demonstrated extraordinary insight and verbal skills and thus enabled a clear presentation of the implementation of self psychology to the treatment of eating disorders.

The first session with Guy and his parents vividly manifested the problematic relationships between the three of them. Guy's father, who experienced himself as lacking emotions, presented Guy with strict demands. He demanded that Guy be the boy that daddy would have wanted him to be. One of the father's demands, raised in therapy, was that Guy develop physical strength and shape. The father mentioned that whenever he was playing soccer with his sons, he would get so focused on the task that he would forget to eat, so the children did not eat either. Guy recalled having to do things for his father because "that's the way it is," with no opportunity to present another opinion or a solution different than the father's. Guy felt that his needs were never acknowledged, let alone legitimated. He felt that he was never given the chance to present his own opinion, never gain recognition and support of his selfhood and thus was never able to develop his distinct identity.

The father's demanding and uncompromising attitude in fact reflected his use of Guy as his selfobject, since Guy served in a role that was his only way to gain recognition. This role was to provide the father with satisfaction and delight and be the son his father managed to shape by his values and perceptions.

Guy's mother was a sensitive, sentimental and vulnerable woman. Her relationship with her husband was unstable, characterized by distance, tensions and a sense of alienation and deprivation. She looked for another partner, another man to support her, soothe her and be there for her to rely on. The chosen partner was Guy.

The family triangle relationship was generated because of the frequent and stressful quarrels between the parents and because the mother turned to Guy for emotional support. Guy recalled a specific quarrel, during a family visit in France, when he heard verbal insults and threats of divorce. After that quarrel, his mother took him for a drive so he would calm her down.

It was therefore evident that not only the father used Guy as his selfobject, but so did the mother. Although the parents seldom agreed with one another, they had implicit agreement to use Guy for their respective selfobject needs.

Guy had difficulties identifying with his rigid and demanding father but identified with his deprived and needy mother. In his relationship with his mother, he found himself in a complicated position: the strong and supportive man on the one hand, and the weak and depressed boy, identifying with the weak and depressed mother, on the other hand. This complicated role, in which weakness and strength, femininity and masculinity, were entangled, made it almost impossible for Guy to develop his own identity. Indeed, as we have seen, Guy stated that he didn't know who he was, or how to grow up.

At initial glance, it seemed that the Oedipal issue was evident in the relationship triangle between Guy and his parents. The Oedipal fantasies aroused by the mother's choice of Guy to help her against her husband might have been the focus of the work at that stage. However, we offered a therapeutic approach that emphasized the importance of the development of the self for Guy, and thus chose not to refer to the Oedipal motive, but only to highlight the theme we found central: the use of Guy as a selfobject, which turned him into a "selfless selfobject" (Goodsitt, 1997).

After the respective use of Guy as a selfobject for each of the parents was discussed in therapy, the parents could recognize their own contribution to establishing this form of relationships with their son. Consequently, they recognized how important it was for them to commence their own therapy where they would discuss their individual and couple issues, thereby making room for their son to live and develop.

At this point, for the first time since Guy began therapy, he was able to perceive himself as someone who can develop and grow, and in the future turn into an adult. He started to discuss his plans to be a musician and an athlete. He also started to express his wish to eat independently, rather than through the feeding tube. At the same time, he expressed great resistance to gaining weight. We interpreted it as a manifestation of his sense of incompetence and littleness, and the accompanying fear that he would have to grow up and undertake duties before he could consolidate his identity and before he feels prepared to go on growing.

The relationship between Guy and his father was central at this phase of therapy. In one session with Guy and his parents, he told his father that he felt that the father was, in Hebrew slang, an "unidentifiable object," a phrase used to designate a person coming from outer space and that he, Guy, did not know him. This opened the discussion of Guy's inability to identify with his father because of his feelings. Guy started gaining weight, which earned him the privilege to go out of the hospital for several hours. In his first time off, he asked to go shopping with his dad, thereby expressing his wish to create a new relationship with his father.

After that point, Guy increasingly expressed other wishes, such as going out of the ward so he could play the guitar. He thus expressed the wish to be allowed to develop his skills and tendencies, to have fun, without suffering. In the music-playing sessions, partially coordinated by the individual therapist, Guy played the guitar skillfully. He described himself as a loser, and while comparing himself to the therapist, idealized the therapist's musical talents. The therapist discussed with him the diversity of people, reflected in their variety of talents, each valuable in itself and worthy of acknowledgment. The therapist pointed out Guy's talent in reading complicated notes, while the therapist was skilled to play by his musical hearing. Guy's talent was not inferior to the therapist's, only different. This was a new concept for Guy, since in his family the attitude to people was only in terms of superiority versus inferiority and success versus failure.

When Guy and the therapist were playing the guitar together, Guy attempted to gain a sense of twinship with the therapist, a constant sense of alikeness, which Kohut (1984) describes as the third selfobject need, along with mirroring and idealization.

Entering the gratifying experience of twinship, while playing music, was difficult for Guy because of his perception of superiority and inferiority. Guy found a way to experience twinship at another level. The therapist was a native English speaker, and at this point of the therapy, Guy started to enjoy speaking English with his therapist, insisting on using English also in the family sessions, despite his parents' poor command of it. These sessions, in which Guy demonstrated his identification with the therapist and idealization of him by using the therapist's mother tongue, expressed the sense of twinship. At the same time, it is possible to interpret his behavior as an act of rebellion against the parents, gaining a sense of superiority over them, and checking their tolerance of his choices, his selfness, even if those are difficult for them.

At this stage, Guy was independently eating all of his meals, gained weight and ceased to talk about death. There were no longer sabotaging behaviors. Now Guy articulated his resistance to his parents watching him in the ward, which we thought was appropriate given his clinical condition. Guy's request attested to progress in therapy, since it signaled Guy's move from his former passive, desperate and destructive position, to an experience of selfness, with developing wishes and skills. He started to take responsibility for his life and to create a broader space for himself. The functioning of the self became more apparent and tangible.

Now, when Guy started to feel that he existed and that this existence was being validated by his surroundings, he began to express his anger toward his family members. One of the things that infuriated him was his parents' change of mind about his weight. In the past, they stressed the importance of thinness and expected him to lose weight. Now, contrary to their previous position, they demand that he gains weight. Discussing this issue, Guy could express his deep experience that he had always served as a selfobject for his family members by "having" to do what they wanted, rather than what he wanted.

Overcoming rupture at this point of therapy highlighted the meaning of selfobject transference evolving between Guy and his therapist. Because of failure to gain weight, the team decided to increase Guy's caloric intake. The decision was implemented, by mistake, before the therapist had a chance to discuss the suggested change with Guy. Guy reacted with fury and with new suicidal threats. We interpreted this harsh response as manifesting Guy's sense of being betrayed by the therapist. Up to that point, Guy perceived his therapist as a reliable selfobject, who always tries to understand Guy's own viewpoint. The intervention here was through adding a session, in which the therapist apologized and admitted it was a mistake not to inform Guy in advance about the planned change. The therapist also referred to the empathic failure that occurred. This intervention soothed Guy and enabled the therapy to go on. Obviously, any therapist in any approach would recognize the mistake and seek to repair it. The emphasis here is that the self psychologically oriented therapist is guided precisely by the meaning attributed to such moments of empathic rupture and failure within self-selfobject relationship. Rupture and reparation within the transference are steps to be crossed for the therapy to progress.

In the last phase of his admission, Guy expressed his disappointment in his failure to gain weight despite his rich meal plan. He began expressing his will to get well and grow up. He talked about a sense of self-identity, and for the first time asked to return home. It was therefore decided to remove his constant watching and allow him to take vacations at home. These changes gave rise to further progress. Guy started to describe better relationship with his father, in which the father's consideration and empathy were evident. Simultaneously, a consistent weight gain resumed, and it was decided to discharge Guy from the hospital.

Guy continued his therapy in a day hospitalization program for three days a week. He returned to his former school a week after his discharge and said that now his first priority was focusing on his studies. He reported how much he enjoyed using his brain and began to read extensively. This behavior reflected the strengthening of his personality and the establishment of motivation.

Guy's integration at school was very successful, and shortly thereafter he asked to discontinue the day hospitalization program so he would not miss school. He asked to continue his therapy only in the outpatient clinic. One day, he refused to finish his meal, ran away and hid in the library. This was interpreted as expressing his wish to be in a place other than the hospital. He still had difficulties expressing his opinions and wishes in words and was forced to express them through avoiding eating, which showed that he deprived himself of a basic need and was harming himself.

It was necessary to respond in therapy. The therapist continued to focus on Guy's will to progress despite the behavior he chose. It was therefore decided to let Guy move to the outpatient clinic, rather than insisting on the day hospitalization program, which would probably be the case had the therapist decided to highlight the need of a more intensive care because of Guy's refusal to eat. Along with discussing Guy's need to express his frustration through self-harm, the therapist focused on Guy's subjective experience that leaving the halfway-out framework meant growth, rather than an interpretation from without seeing it solely as resistance.

Guy's first request in the outpatient clinic was to gain more privacy. He felt that his parents received too much information from the therapist. This request demonstrated the development of Guy's self-definition, which became increasingly cohesive, and the emergence of a new will to establish more appropriate boundaries. Guy's request was approved. Psychotherapy now began to discuss Guy's relationship with his mother, including Guy's need of a psychic space that would be free of her. Guy raised the question whether it was possible to distinguish self-image from weight. This question reflected Guy's identification with his mother, who translated her own self-image to focusing on her weight, as well as his attempt to break free of such heritage of low self-esteem.

As Guy was approaching his target weight, he frequently spoke on his "deep deep down" wish to heal. Alongside this wish, he also felt fear. He talked about still feeling the need to rely on his illness and to look ill, and in fact it was hard for him to feel that he had any identity outside the ill one: "Who am I if I am not an anorexic?" The following dialogue illustrates the therapeutic approach used in this situation. The therapist aligned with Guy's subjective experience and validated the existence and legitimacy of his healthy self, thereby allowing a change in Guy's self-image.

Guy: Deep deep down I want to heal completely, but I still don't want to eat spontaneously. Sometimes I still want to be viewed as ill. I need to be different.

Therapist: What do you make of it?

G: I guess it makes me feel good.

T: You rely on food instead of feeling that you have an identity, it is as if the illness became your identity.

G: Yes, it's true that I don't feel like I have an identity. I don't feel special beyond this.

T: I believe you have an identity. You still feel unworthy, not existing, without the illness's uniqueness, but from our long acquaintance I know you are very special beyond your illness.

After several months of therapy in the outpatient clinic, Guy reached his target weight. He managed to eat out in a restaurant and declared: "I think I don't need the food stuff anymore." He described his future plans, which included his aspiration to go to a boarding high school. It was at this time that a change appeared in his behavior both at home and in his social interactions. He started to stand up for his rights and assertively protect his possessions, both at home and outside. For example, when the family met financial troubles and had to sell some valuables, Guy refused to allow the sale of beloved belongings. Referring to this situation, he stated that now he "lived for himself," therefore he also took care of his belongings. The therapist validated Guy's right to be strong and stand up for himself.

From a self psychology perspective, Guy's statements pointed to a significant structural shift in his self. Whereas previously Guy was a selfless selfobject (Goodsitt, 1997), felt worthless and unable to advance his interests and growth, now he began to highlight his place and his status in the world.

At this stage, Guy was struggling to define his "life objective." He said in this regard that there wasn't any *one* that he loved, but he was able to love a dog. He felt that it was easier to love a dog, since "a dog won't hate you, won't harm you, will always be with you and do whatever *you* want." This fantasy of a dog serving as his selfobject and meeting his needs expressed the wish that his parents failed to realize. Up to this point, Guy turned to food for selfobject functions because he was frustrated when his parents and other people could not meet these needs for him (Sands, 1989, 1991). Now he turned to a living selfobject, however not human – a dog. This was a crucial step in the development of his self and in his healing process. It signaled progress from turning to inanimate selfobject, like food, to a living selfobject, even if this selfobject had less autonomy than a human being.

In light of these developments, the focus in therapy around the time Guy returned home was to help his parents provide him with more selfobject functions. Thus, for example, his mother received help to allow him a larger emotional space rather than use him as a selfobject by being consoled by him when sad. His father needed assistance to show more interest in Guy's viewpoint in their talks and to be able to understand Guy's perspective. Guy felt better at home (after previously saying "it ain't my home!"), for instance when his father played soccer with him. In therapy, Guy expressed a wish that joint activities with his father would also be at the father's initiative, not only at his own (the therapist told the father about this wish). Guy wanted his father to be interested in him and wish to be in his company. The inner questions emerging here are "am I worthy of others, especially of my parents?" and "do they want to be with *me* for who *I am*?"

Guy started to inquire about the therapist's feelings for him and wondered how it was possible for the therapist to "love" more than one patient. The following dialogue illustrates the emphasis put by the therapist on Guy's uniqueness.

G: Do you ever think about your patients?

T: It seems to me that you are asking whether I think about you, whether you mean something for me. I think you know that you do.

G: Have you worked with someone else for a longer time [than you did with me]?

T: You want to know how you are compared to my other patients; whether you are special to me or just another patient. I think these questions emerge because you lack the feeling that you are special for who you are, that you can be loved for who you are. You still feel you can be loved only if you fulfill the needs of someone else.

G: Right. I have always lived for others. I did everything for others. I want to live *my* life. [At this point in therapy Guy refers to the increasing recognition that he had to meet his father's expectations regardless of his own aspirations, and he was more aware of his mother's lack of boundaries in their emotional relationships.]

T: You lack the feeling that you are special on your own account.

G: I don't lack it, it does not exist. When you don't have something, you don't lack it. It's like computers one hundred years ago, when they didn't have computers yet. Did anyone lack it?

In this session, we discussed Guy's lack of self-experience and turning to a human figure (the therapist) through transference of his wish for a selfobject. Perhaps Guy's interest in the therapist's feelings (indeed feelings for him) signals another progress in therapy. Guy allows himself to view his therapist as an object with his own interests and feelings, which indicates development in the consolidation of his self. Mirroring his needs of acknowledgment and of feeling special helped Guy, over time, to feel more comfortable, to acknowledge his uniqueness and recognize his talents. Guy realized that "self-image is in fact self-satisfaction, rather than the satisfaction of others." He expressed his wish to "realize the self to the fullest." These statements were living evidence for the development of a self-structure after Guy was released from the position of fulfilling others' selfobject needs.

Guy's experience of "selflessness" stemmed both from the fact he had to fulfill his parents' selfobject needs and the fact that he never gained their support for developing his sense of self. Because of his parents' failure to satisfy his selfobject needs, Guy turned to food (or to avoiding it) to meet these needs. Guy had to protect this substitute "like a man protects a part of his self" (Sands, 1989). Guy's depression, suicidal intentions and anger may be perceived as expressions of the threat of disintegration he experienced at the time, and of the deprivation of selfobject he needed.

The task in therapy was to develop a self-structure within Guy, which would enable him to regulate his emotions and soothe himself by himself. The road to this objective goes through the ability to use a human figure to fulfill selfobject needs instead of substance – food.

The more the therapist could be experienced as a reliable selfobject and focused on Guy's subjective experience, his legitimate narcissistic tendencies and his needs, the more Guy could heal, and his need to starve himself will decrease. The experience that he doesn't have to serve as a selfobject for the therapist but rather the therapist serves as a selfobject for him was novel to him. In the past, he felt like living in a "script," in which he had to please his parents and perform the role they expected of him. The opportunity to idealize the therapist in the transference (at one point Guy said, "I bet you get along with everyone!"), to receive his mirroring of his selfobject needs and awareness of empathic failures, enabled Guy to turn to other human beings to fulfill basic needs of the self instead of turning to an inanimate substance. Simultaneously,

Guy's parents were able to begin and satisfy Guy's selfobject needs such as expressing more interest in his wishes and aspirations, and a willingness to respect them, which, for example, was practically demonstrated when they bought him a dog. By this Guy's self was released from its developmental arrest, and development of a healthier and more cohesive self became possible.

9 A Journey to the Inner Core

Myrna Milun

Noa, a young single woman aged 23, Israeli-born, a first-year art student, presented for treatment at the eating disorders outpatient clinic at Hadassah University Hospital in Jerusalem.

She reported binge eating and purging that had begun approximately five years before. The frequency of bingeing and purging ranged from a few times a day to a few times a week. Her "struggle with food," as she put it, was a "central pillar" in her life. She felt unable to cope with day-to-day activities and decisions. She reported fluctuating mood states, lack of self-confidence and poor self and body image. It was her perception that "Bad Noa eats forbidden foods without control and Good Noa eats appropriate foods in small portions and with control." She was diagnosed with bulimia nervosa.

Noa had previously been in therapy three times but had terminated after a few months at most.

She appears somewhat younger than her 23 years. She has an average build and pleasant appearance. She dresses fashionably, often with one eye-catching accessory. She is highly intelligent. Her vocabulary is rich and her discourse is often interwoven with "psychological insights" probably acquired in previous treatments. She speaks continuously during the therapeutic hour, moving frenetically from topic to topic. Her mood is often dysphoric. She expresses much frustration with her life, appears distressed and is usually disconnected from her emotions.

Noa is the second daughter in a family of three girls, residing in a community village in the South of Israel. Her father, a physician, is described as a tough and demanding person who she feels always pressures her to achieve more, while she describes him as a failure, "a deflated human being" and regards him as immature and irresponsible. She describes their relationship as one of love-hate. The mother is a librarian. Noa reports her relationship with her as very close and special; however she does not describe it in any clear terms. She describes her mother's need to be with her and know her innermost thoughts – "mom cannot live without me." Noa hints at underlying stresses in her relationship with her older sister and only seldom mentions her younger sister.

Noa describes having a happy childhood. Things went well for her. She was the "queen" of the class. Yet, there was always a feeling lurking below the surface of a lack of fulfillment or satisfaction. A dramatic turning point came when Noa was 15. Her mother was diagnosed with severe kidney failure and underwent surgery and dialysis. The trauma was not worked through in the family at all. A year later, her father was facing serious financial problems. Noa learned that she needed to take care of herself and rely only on herself. Not long after this, she began to perceive herself as fat. Upon graduating from high school, she performed two years of mandatory military service. During this time, she began to feel an emptiness, which she "filled" with bingeing and purging. She hid her symptoms from family and friends – "they did not see."

After her army service, she worked for a while and then travelled abroad. She felt cut off from the world, irritable and aggressive toward others and lacked self-confidence. It was while abroad that she first approached therapy.

Noa had several relationships with young men, all of which are described as complicated and frustrating. She has many girlfriends with whom she has rather intense relationships.

Noa is gifted with artistic talents but describes great frustration in her art studies. There, as in other areas of her life, she appears to be striving for a perfect ideal and is disappointed in herself and her surroundings time and again.

She was diagnosed as suffering from bulimia nervosa with narcissistic personality traits. It was decided to see her for long-term psychotherapy, once a week.

Already in the very first therapy session, Noa brought up a vague description out of which the therapist was able to see the correlation between feeling rejected and empty and the urge to binge. She had some idea that her eating behavior expressed psychological tensions. She expressed little faith in psychotherapy but felt that a treatment program including medical and nutritional care, as was provided in our clinic, was necessary. In the past, "things did not connect" in therapy, she said. She never experienced satisfaction. She was jealous of others who had a significant and satisfying relationship. She expressed self-loathing and the desire to be someone else. She described emptiness and an inability to be creative, to make decisions and to make an effort. She also described her need to protect her mother, not to cause her worry. She claimed that her family and friends did not notice her bingeing and purging. She spoke of social activities where others had not succeeded in reaching her in an emotional sense, had not known who she really was.

In the initial sessions, Noa described the week's events in a frenetic fashion that was nonetheless quite disconnected from emotions. She jumped from one event to another and back again, filled the room with words and left the therapist with no time to respond and no opportunity to recall the sequence of the sessions in a logical way.

The bingeing disappeared after the first month of therapy, and there began a process of seeing the bulimia as a symptom of something else, and a process of identifying her emotions. In the absence of binges, Noa experienced great difficulty in finding a focus both in her life and in therapy. She felt "fragmented." In the sixth session, she reported being with her mother and yet feeling alone; something was there between them that could not be touched. In this session, she reported events in an emotionally disconnected fashion. The therapist was able to point this out and show how she had expected a warm hug from her mother but had felt unable to request one. She was left with a silent and empty space, and in fact, was deeply disappointed with her mother's emotional response to her. In the following session, she reported having had a wave of purging and said she had "broken all the rules." She had attempted to explain to her mother the insights of the previous session but had not succeeded in doing so very clearly, nor in getting across the intensity of the session's emotional impact. Her mother strongly rejected Noa's interpretation of the events. Noa reported other interactions that had left her feeling empty, after which she ate chocolate and vomited.

The sequence was becoming clearer. Then followed a month with no significant progress. Working through connections between dysphoric emotions and bingeing and purging continued thereafter. It is important to note that this "bingeing" was on a far smaller scale; in fact, it consisted of eating the "wrong" foods, according to Noa's rules, not to any real excess.

Noa began to discuss her difficulties in coping with projects at art school. She understood that she was required to express her inner being and felt unable to connect with this inner core. She was terrified that there was nothing there. She felt like a filthy garbage bin from the inside. The therapist showed her that at certain times in her life, when it had been very hard for her, there was no one there for her. She had lacked someone who would admire and show interest in her inner being. Thus, she buried it down deep, never showed it on the outside and secretly purged.

She began to cry for the first time in the therapy, which had now been in progress for three months. She brought her own examples of her parents' lack of adequate emotional attunement to her. Gradually, she was able to bring examples of the need to eat "forbidden" foods (binge-triggering foods) and vomit in response to feelings of rejection, jealousy and emptiness.

The therapist repeatedly identified Noa's experiences of lack of confirmation, failures in empathy and others' lack of attunement to her needs while asserting their own needs. Time after time, the therapist reflected Noa's need to satisfy the needs of her mother and her friends. Noa had difficulty in adopting this interpretation but gradually became convinced. Concomitant with this progress, order and logical cohesion emerged in Noa's self-presentation, improving the therapist's ability to record the sessions.

Noa began to report incidents of dysphoria in which she had managed not to vomit. In the fifteenth session, she reported telling a friend she needed her and thinking that the therapist would be pleased. She had decided to go on a trip to South America for the summer, which meant a three-month break from the therapy. In the session before the break, she again returned to the disjointed mode as seen in the initial stage. She referred to her lack of faith in the therapy at the beginning and compared it with her present feeling that she could not cope without it. She requested a coping device from the therapist. The therapist suggested she listen to her bulimic part, to try to understand the needs expressed by that part of herself and look for alternative ways of satisfying those needs.

When Noa returned from her trip, she reported several incidents of other people rejecting her, and consequent feelings of loneliness, lack of self-worth and emptiness, which in turn led to "unhealthy" eating behavior. Her introspection and insight began to take on new depth. She was able to see disparate attributes in herself. She described the feeling of intense excitement during a philosophy lecture where she felt connected with her innermost being. On the other hand, however, a while later, she felt completely fragmented because of a single word said to her by her older sister.

Noa reported a continuous search for herself at art school. We talked about her difficulty to connect with this inner core without appropriate acknowledgment from the outside. In this context, we discussed her mother's use of her as a selfobject. We recalled her conversation with her mother on the eve of her departure to South America. Her mother again told her that she could not live without her, which Noa took as a sign of her mother's closeness to her. The therapist showed Noa how this was an expression of her mother's anxiety, without acknowledging Noa's need to separate and embark upon a voyage that was part of her search for herself. The following session showed some regression to disjointedness and pathological eating behavior. Noa yearned to be understood by others without any struggle on her part. A few sessions later, she described how someone unexpectedly helped her and her subsequent feeling of being energized. A former boyfriend rejected her and she felt empty, but she was able to ask a friend for support and to explain her feelings and needs. This experience was also revitalizing.

She then went headlong into an intimate relationship with a young man she wanted even though she understood he was not able to genuinely give of himself. She was able to actively overcome several insults within this relationship. Despite pressure at art school, she did not feel empty and did not turn to food for self-soothing. For the first time since starting therapy nine months before, she reported feeling optimistic.

Within a short time, she saw that she could not maintain this stance over a long period. A disappointment from the relationship gave rise to symptoms and she considered giving up the relationship to preserve normal eating. The therapist pointed out how food still seemed more reliable than people. Some criticism leveled against her at school had a similar effect. The therapist helped her understand that she was offended because the teacher and the other students had not been able to see her work from her point of view.

The relationship with the young man was short-lived. Noa was able to express her anger at his inability to give any place to her feelings. Her ability to identify what hurt her in his attitude was a sign of considerable progress, but she was still hurt by his lack of acknowledgment of her feelings and symptoms returned. Noa understood the emotional sequence but was not able to stop the process. After a while, she reported a family meeting in which she felt cared for by her family, which enabled her to avoid vomiting although she had eaten a large amount. She suffered another rejection from a young man but did not "fall apart" because she received support from her girlfriends. She felt able to deal with the pressures at school and reported having successfully expressed something of herself in her artwork.

At this point, we delved into the parallel process of her search for her inner self, both in her artistic work and in the therapy. She reported being good at sketching where there was less call for expression of her inner self.

In the thirtieth session, she reported in great detail on a project in which she had invested much energy. She had worked on it day and night, felt a sense of accomplishment and success both in the work and in the presentation and enjoyed the process of creation. She was required to design an accessory and decided on a head covering. She created it in the shape of a tulip, partly closed in front and open at the back. The frontal closure signified her need to look inwards and cut herself off from her surroundings, so as not to be permanently activated by and responsive to others' behavior toward her. The anterior opening and other small openings still allowed some external influence. The object was aesthetically pleasing, the work very precise. For Noa, this was proof that she was still too involved with externalities and the impression she made on others. She felt that she stood behind this project in a novel way, in a manner that she had not felt previously in her studies. She felt she had reached a milestone even though she had not yet attained her final goal. During the work on this project, she felt that the class worked closely together and that more meaningful connections were formed with her fellow students than she had experienced previously. She said that in this project, she had managed "to put herself aside." The therapist interpreted that she had been less self-conscious and more open and available to her surrounding and her work and could be more spontaneous in the creative process.

We discussed the disparate parts of herself and her difficulty in integrating them. For example, a "child" part, impulsive and irresponsible, as opposed to an "adult" part, ambitious, mature, serious and goal oriented. She reported receiving feedback at art school that a former presentation was too black and white. There was no gray. She said how much she disliked the color gray, and the symbolism was not lost on her.

Not only in her artwork was there an expression of inner introspection, Noa enthusiastically participated in a course given by a rabbi. She often felt that he was speaking directly to her and was frequently brought to tears in his lectures. In a specific lecture, the rabbi referred to Rabbi Kook and his perception of the Jewish nation as being divided into two group – the people of "chaos," and the people of "reparation." Noa felt that she belonged to the people of "chaos," people without a clear framework, without rules, who search for their own independent way. And even though this way is more difficult, they are able to reach greater heights. She felt, however, that she also possessed a few features of the "reparation" group. This confused her. The therapist pointed out her complexity of character, that she did not belong entirely to one side of a dichotomy, namely, that there was no black and white.

A change of the therapist's weekly schedule disrupted the continuity of weekly meetings, causing the cancellation of one therapy session once a month. Noa expressed her dissatisfaction with the changes, and the therapist acknowledged her response. Noa was able to express more optimism that there was indeed a central core to herself. She described successfully overcoming the desire to vomit while she was alone by telling herself that in a few hours she would feel differently and there would be no more need. In addition, she understood that had a friend been there with her, she would not have been able to or need to purge. Noa could cope with both positive and negative feedback from others.

These feelings reflected a process of transmuting internalization, in which Noa discovered her own propensity for self-regulation and self-soothing, functions that had been previously provided by the therapist. Noa feared that her anchoring points were too fragile and that she might lose them too easily. She was concerned about her lack of focus, concentration, internal organization and connectedness. We discussed how she desired experience to fill her up as if she were an empty tank.

Noa reported a conversation with her mother about a past mutual experience where she had not felt understood. She explained to her mother that she would have liked her to have seen, accepted and given more room to her emotions. She was able to express criticism of her family and their way of communicating. Symptom-wise, she felt she could give up the binges but not the vomiting.

At this point, the strike of the clinical psychologists in the public sector in Israel forced the therapist to temporarily halt the therapy. In self psychology terms, a massive, nationwide empathic failure was perpetrated. In a phone call, the therapist divulged to Noa that she was writing this case report. Noa felt important to the therapist, that she had a special place in her heart and mind. In this way, she was able to overcome the long break in the therapy.

After a three-month break, the therapeutic sessions were resumed. Noa experienced the therapist as an empathic figure, and in her absence was able to develop the seeds of self-care through transmuting internalization.

Noa reported that food was no longer an issue in her life and that she was no longer bulimic. She had not believed she could reach this stage. She had attained her goal weight without dieting.

Now Noa was preoccupied with the give and take of relationships, with envy of others possessing traits that she lacked and with the desire for a permanent intimate relationship, which would provide her with on tap empathy and mirroring. She strongly felt that she was always in someone else's "script," fulfilling his needs, with no "script" of her own. She constantly checked whether others were considerate of her needs, whether they treated her favorably and whether they were attentive. The therapist interpreted that she was hungry for contact, for confirmation from others in place of food. The search was still not balanced, a little desperate, too needy, somewhat "bulimic." Noa understood that if she felt basic acceptance by someone, she would be able to overcome little insults or lapses in empathy on the part of that person.

In her talks with her family, she expected more emotional involvement on their part and tried to educate them with her newly discovered insights gained from the therapy. We deepened our understanding of the family dynamics. Noa described in detail the differences between her and her older sister. Her sister was organized, ambitious, serious and an achiever. Noa, the cute, free-spirited one, was none of these things. The therapist suggested that each one had found a special place in their parents' hearts and because, at certain times, they had not had much space to offer, it was forbidden for one sister to take up the special space reserved for her sister. Thus, they had developed totally different characteristics; and it had become very difficult for Noa to adopt behaviors characteristic of her sister and difficult to become more whole. It appeared that the times when Noa felt her parents to have the least space available and the scarcest resources to give were the times of crisis for the parents. Indeed, the parents had been poorly able to attend to their daughter's viewpoint all along, but at the time of the mother's illness or the father's financial difficulties, neither of them was available to make up for the other's unavailability.

While discussing a crisis with a friend, caused by Noa's prolonged denial of her own needs in favor of her friend's needs, we approached the origin of this behavioral pattern. Noa found great difficulty in being critical of her mother and the therapist interpreted that this difficulty pointed to her inability to see her from a distance, from the standpoint of separation. Noa's mother could not feel good if Noa did not feel good. She felt bad if Noa told her that she was stressed or tired, causing Noa to feel guilty that she had burdened her mother with her feelings. Noa did not allow herself the right to feel her own feelings and she had not allowed herself any adolescent rebellion against her parents, making room for separation.

Noa still feared somewhat that she could not be creative from within. The therapist encouraged her that now, when she was not so involved with food, she was more available and internally organized. Noa reported that she had successfully made the "right connections" in her art school project, communicated herself clearly and received good critical feedback. At her final project presentation that year, she felt more confident in herself, in her creative ability and in her ability to express herself. She was able to dramatically impress the lecturer and fellow students with her work. She was filled with the joy of living and felt she possessed the strength to create, to be assertive and to be there for her friends. There were no more extreme mood fluctuations or the confused self-presentation. In their place were signs of self-cohesion and of inner strength. The end of therapy was in sight. It continued for an additional year of successful consolidation work.

Some years later, on a visit to the hospital for a different medical issue, Noa contacted the therapist. She reported that she had been symptom-free since the termination of therapy and that she was happily married with three children and had designed a product that she sold in a successful self-owned business.

Noa's therapy highlights some central issues relating to self psychology's perception of eating disorders. Sands (1991) sees the disordered mind's dissociations a major focal point for therapy. Noa displayed significant dissociative elements that were reflected in her disconnected initial self-presentation, the splits in her personality, her emotional disconnectedness and hints of what Sands (1991) names the "bulimic self."

The therapist's difficulty in finding and following a main theme in Noa's frenetic talk was described earlier. There was a sense of fragmentation in the initial stages of therapy. Recognizing the empathic failure Noa experienced, along with the empathic atmosphere in therapy, allowed the development of a more cohesive self-presentation.

Noa manifested many occurrences of dissociation. In the first sessions, she talked about "Good Noa and Bad Noa." She felt immense disparity between her actual self and her ideal self. The actual self had a sense of emptiness, but she aspired wholeness, creation and harmony. She often described opposing characteristics of herself. She was "queen of the class" or the opposite, critical, distanced, rejecting others. Sometimes she could give to others, sometimes she could not. She was indifferent and reserved, or on the contrary, overwhelmed with emotions, enthusiastic or highly distressed. She was a perfectionist or someone who could not make an effort – a disorganized procrastinator. She sought depth and power or she was superficial and sought easy and immediate solutions. She was a careful planner or the opposite, careless and haphazard. She was strong and alternatively weak, fragile and fragmented. Taken together, all these elements highlighted her lack of self-cohesiveness.

At the beginning of therapy, Noa manifested emotional disconnectedness – she described events in an intellectual manner and with no emotions. This was particularly evident when she described interactions with her mother. For a long time, she was not able to spontaneously describe emotions related to her mother.

According to Sands (1991), the central dissociative element is the patient's bulimic self. Sands describes it as a dissociated part that contains the archaic selfobject needs that were repressed and channeled into the eating disorder. Noa named her bulimic self "Bad Noa who lost control." It took a long time to help her listen to this part inside her. Only after many months of therapy was she able to accept this part, confirm it and acknowledge its positive traits; namely, to begin to integrate this part into her personality. It is Sands's contention that this process is facilitated by the therapist's attempts to mirror both sides of the split, to explain them as two different coping strategies and "hold" the entire patient at once.

Another manifestation of Noa's disconnection from herself was found in her difficulty to find a core in her artwork, to connect with her inner self and to find a genuine expression of her central core. The therapeutic process was an attempt to find her true self. We often discussed the parallel between her development at art school and her development in therapy, as detailed previously.

The integration of dissociated parts and the process of transmuting internalization provide for the ability to more efficiently use narcissistic energies and channel them for creation (Kohut, 1971).

Another key element in Noa's therapy is her use of food instead of people to fulfill selfobject needs (Goodsitt, 1985; Sands, 1991). The development of this process is parallel to the development of the bulimic self. The case report abounds with examples of bingeing and purging as a reaction to experiences of rejection, emptiness and empathic failure. Noa gradually developed the ability to identify the emotional motives of her behavior and to perceive her bulimia as a symptom of something deeper. She began to recognize empathic failures toward her on the part of other people, or their use of her as selfobject.

Gradually, the bulimic symptoms diminished. Noa began the slow and painful process of turning to other people to satisfy her selfobject needs, and she started to relate to empathic failure on the part of the therapist, although the transference was seldom analyzed. This is in accordance with Kohut's (1987a) suggestion that in the treatment of patients with severe disorders of the self, a very long phase is needed to be devoted to empathic understanding and mirroring, without interpretations. According to Bollas (1987), such patients typically ignore the interpretation's content because of their exclusive need for an empathic atmosphere in therapy, which is "the constant song of the analytic voice."

10 I Am Not Allowed to Be a Whole Person

Varda Shavit Ohayon

Moranne, a 24-year-old law student, was referred to psychotherapy by her metabolic doctor who diagnosed a continuous deterioration of her restrictive type anorexia. When she entered therapy, she weighed 37 kg and her height was 1.68 m. She was living with a boyfriend at the time. The severe deterioration began two years earlier, when she lost over 10 kg of her weight. It started after breaking up with a former boyfriend. "He was my first boyfriend. I cried my eyes out, I was desperate. I went on tough diets. I loved starving myself, I felt masochistic. Anyway since my birth I thought life was meant to suffer in it." Moranne was obsessively and cruelly preoccupied with physical exercise. "I was calculating when I would return home so I could abuse myself." Moranne felt an inner urge to perform these exercises to lose weight, even though they caused her pain. Sometimes she felt fear when she woke up in the morning because she knew she would have to perform them. She always felt she could not enjoy life and that life wasn't meant for joy but instead to fulfill others' expectations of her.

At the first stage of therapy, Moranne tells me about her obsessive preoccupation with food. She is happy when she is hungry. If she eats, she becomes terrified that she might never be hungry again. If she eats something during the day not in the presence of her close ones, she feels anxiety and guilt. Her hunger and eating with her close ones are the presents she gives them. If it was the case that she ate by herself during the day, then she'd perform difficult physical activities: walking instead of taking the bus or climbing up the stairs. She would not be at peace "until the last drop of sugar leaves my body." Her obsessive preoccupation with food causes her pain and she feels crazy and masochistic. In the therapy room, she sets her eyes on a book titled "Denying Death" and asks if it is about people like her. Moranne hates the time she spends in the university. These are the times when she is by herself. She wants to eat, but when she is alone, she feels she cannot do it, as if she cannot live, exist and enjoy herself if it is for herself and not for someone else. She feels she cannot share her pain with her parents or her boyfriend.

At this stage of therapy, Moranne does not gain weight, does not follow the nutritionist's instructions and even appears to lose weight. One session I offer her a candy I have in my bag. I am doubtful whether I am cautious enough not to get involved or put too much pressure on her. We eat the candies together. She understands that I want to actually see what it is all about. She eats the candy as if she swallows a bitter pill – with rigid and stiff mouth movement as if she cannot let the sweetness touch her. Nonetheless, she experiences my offer as an actual interest in her rather than an attempt to baby-feed her. At this point, after she describes a day of self-torture at the university, I tell Moranne that I see she is feeling as if it is forbidden for her to be a whole human being – a human being who wants things as she pleases and in her own time and who satisfies herself when she wants something. Apparently, this intervention is highly meaningful for her. She returns to it and recites it frequently in other sessions. She says she indeed feels like she cannot let herself be a whole person. After this therapeutic work, she tries to eat by herself and describes candidly how anxious it made her, how hard it is for her to eat for herself rather for someone else and how she is filled with a desire to annihilate what her body has absorbed by choice. It is as if she seeks to eliminate any evidence that she has needs and that she satisfies them. At this time in therapy, when it is hard for her to exit sessions that were meaningful and gratifying for her, she says, "You probably don't have time for me."

The second stage of therapy seems to have conflicting wishes of separation, self-definition and autonomy. She says, "If I was on a desert island I would be healed." She feels that when she is away from her significant others and from their expectations, she will be able to let herself heal and sense her selfhood. Alongside these wishes, she brings up wishes to regain increasing independence, and she is angry with herself because of her constant effort to please others. She learns, in therapy, that she used to look for others' wishes and intensify them within herself even when those wishes were scarce and weak. Thus, for example, she feels obligated to clean her mother's house even when it is doubtful whether the mother actually asked for it, and although in retrospect her mother clearly gave it up. She needs and asks for approval to be able to want for herself and do for herself. She tells me that at home she told her father: "Hug me, tell me I am allowed to eat."

In the third stage of therapy, Moranne examines her relationship with her boyfriend. She links her need to please and not disappoint and her fear that he would not want her if she behaves differently. She recalls former relationships, in which she also experienced a strong fear of being abandoned. She recalls a relationship with a boy who "was really gross" but she dated him because she felt unworthy. She angrily remembers that her mother pushed her to date this guy explaining to her that there isn't always love at first sight. It is as if her mother, too, is not sure that Moranne would be desirable. At this point, Moranne examines the extent of satisfaction in her current relationship. She is afraid that even today she may find herself doing things that do not cause her happiness. Thus, for instance, she describes her responsiveness to sex as not being connected to her passion but to her obedience because her boyfriend "needs to get what he wants." Under the therapy's wings, Moranne attempts to be more frank and determined at home and in her relationship with her boyfriend. To her surprise, she discovers that when she has "more body" (by that she means a bigger presence), fears of her boyfriend come up that she may want to leave him. It never occurred to her before that someone may actually fear being left by her, and she finds it amusing. Simultaneously, Moranne gains weight, and when she crosses significant lines, like the 40 kg line, she announces them excitedly.

In the fourth stage, Moranne reports better and happier days on the one hand, but days of depression and lack of energy on the other hand. She is afraid that her diligence, which was associated with perfectionism and will to please others, is being substituted by laziness and weakness. She cries a lot. She decides to get married, and she is happy and confident about the relationship, but is afraid that she is entering prison. The certain autonomy she gained is not experienced as completely stable and natural. She eats nice amounts of food and even enjoys food. She is less preoccupied with the obsessive thinking around food, but then she fears she might lose control and never stop eating. At this point, the fragility of her sense of autonomy is highly evident: Is it possible to preserve this sense and still feel intimacy? Will she need to go everywhere with her husband from now on?

After a year of therapy, we prepared to end it. I left my work at the clinic and Moranne got married and found a job in a Southern village, far away from Jerusalem. In the final session, she brought her wedding album. In the photos and in real life she looked happy and healthy. Moranne and her parents expressed both orally and in writing deep gratitude for their sense that her life was saved. I replied, and I sincerely believe it, that recovery was made possible because of Moranne's will and persistence in therapy, and thanks to her will to choose life. After her weight and menstruation were found normal in follow-ups, she could terminate metabolic follow-ups as well.

I think that if asked, Moranne would say that the central message she held onto in the therapy was that "she is allowed to be herself." In psychotherapy language, she would probably mean the message of approval and acknowledgment of her selfhood. The strongest insight that Moranne felt in therapy was, I think, when she understood how strong her sense was that she is not allowed to be a whole person who chooses to enjoy life, to exist and to be present. Concretely speaking, the change she underwent was that prior to the treatment she felt that if she was eating not for another person, it is as if she was eating against this person; and after the treatment, she understood that she is allowed to eat also for herself and to satisfy her own needs.

11 Satiable Hunger

Sara Haramati

Shani reached the hospital suffering from severe anorexia nervosa, restrictive type. Her weight was 15 kg lower than the desired weight, she was exhausted and dehydrated and it was clear that she would need immediate hospitalization. Shani responded to the admission decision with passive acceptance, almost relief.

Through her therapy, Shani managed to recover from her eating disorder and achieve considerable improvement of her mental health, functioning and feelings.

Shani is the second daughter of a father who is a lawyer and a mother who is a housewife. She says that her mother was deeply connected to Shani's older brother and adored him; while all Shani got from her was criticism and a sense of disappointment. As a child, she kept hearing how the neighborhood's children were more beautiful and successful than her. The father, she says, was always busy in work and wasn't attentive to his children's needs.

Upon her admission, it turned out that Shani has been trying to lose weight since her early adolescence. She was anorexic at some points, and bulimic at others. When she graduated from high school she was enlisted to the army, where her condition deteriorated – she ate less and less and performed more and more physical exercise. The adults around her, both at home and in the army, hardly saw what was going on with her and certainly did not know how to intervene. Only after several months, when Shani's physical condition became acutely severe, were her parents forced to realize her condition; and even at that point, Shani was reluctant to agree and accept their intervention.

Her father managed to bring her to our unit only through a "deal" he made with her: he "arranged" for an army discharge, on non-psychiatric grounds, in exchange for her consent to accept therapy. It later turned out that it was the first time ever that her father joined the treatment efforts, and apparently it was also a significant factor in her consent.

On Shani's part, her hospital admission was a stark turning point: years of uninterrupted self-harm and disordered eating, with no adult around her aware or able to intervene, were abruptly brought to an end. The experience of being alone with her destructive behaviors – unaccountable for herself or others regarding her actions and reasons – was radically changed here. At the hospital, she had dramatically less control over her activity. The nurses watched her during each meal and between meals; she was forbidden from leaving the ward, and visits had to follow a pre-arranged plan; psychotherapy – which she previously refused – constituted a central part of the plan.

Her hospital caretakers stressed the message that the most important goals were to protect her health and nutrition and to prevent her from self-harm. Anything that was first priority for Shani thus far – being thin and depriving herself of virtually any basic need – was now defined as conflicting with her best interest and her real needs. She was told in so many ways that she did not and probably could not succeed in taking care of herself, so the staff would undertake that task.

In therapy, she was told the following:

> You are like a pilot in a state of vertigo. In this situation, if the pilot follows her instincts, she'd crash. She must obey the control tower's commands. We are the control tower, and you must follow our orders in order to avoid crashing.

For Shani, this was an entirely new experience of "being seen" and mirrored in the eyes of parental adults who see her, see her needs and want to take care of her. These adults perceive their role, at this initial stage, as fulfilling the functions she is not able to fulfill herself. This experience was created in two different care levels: One level was inpatient case management – feeding, watching, setting boundaries – which all provided Shani with a sense of protection and genuine attention to *her* needs. A second level was psychotherapy. When the physical aspects were properly taken care of, space was created for psychotherapeutic exploration and observation. In the sessions, Shani talked about herself, her childhood experiences, her feelings and her thoughts. With time, a picture emerged of a girl abandoned by her parents in everything that had to do with emotional parental functions. It seemed that the mother treated her children very differently: Shani's brother was contained in the maternal symbiosis and symboled anything the mother considered admirable and gratifying; whereas the rejected and disappointing parts were projected onto Shani. Shani painfully recalled countless examples of her mother's mirroring, from teasing and humiliating nicknames to responses like "beautiful?

Come on!" when Shani was complimented by others. Shani also found it difficult to forgive her father, who refrained from taking part in this drama through retreating to his work and private world.

Thanks to talking about herself and the positive mirroring provided by the therapist, Shani began to recognize the connection between her self-starvation and her prolonged emotional hunger. Gradually, she started to feel that avoiding food, which she used to consider remarkable self-control, was in fact severe dysfunction. She hoped that the pursuit of thinness would serve to establish a sense of specialty and identity but realized that it was in fact destroying her.

Thus, by responding to therapy, Shani could delegate to others control over fulfilling some of her needs and begin to feel the pleasure and comfort it entails: over the following months, this basic need that had been deprived for years, was beginning to get satisfied. The inevitable weight gains are now little less terrifying. Healthy eating – however still rigid and entirely planned – became bearable, although not enjoyable yet.

Progress inescapably brought about getting ready for discharge from the hospital, and a question was raised concerning going back home. Discussing the issue in therapy, it became clear that Shani could not go back there: the opportunity she was given by the staff to reject her mother's visits made her feel supported and protected. In the few meetings that did take place between Shani and her mother, Shani discovered that the old experiences are repeated time and again: she feels that her mother does not contain her and rejects her. Touching upon those experiences and working them through did not lead to reconciliation and understanding, but only to Shani's desire to distance herself from her mother. Her father, on the contrary, was more actively engaged in therapy than his previous participation in his daughter's life up to that point, thus earned himself a significant role in Shani's new life. Shani could work through her disappointments of him and accept him with all his limitations. This state of affairs also provided the solution to the discharge dilemma: it was decided that Shani would move to a rented apartment and that her father would provide for her rent and expenses. This solution, in which her father was "holding" her financially and emotionally the best he could, allowed Shani to leave the hospital's protection, while still feeling protected and not feeling abandoned. She designed a situation in which she assumes those self-functions she was able to fulfill by herself but also relies on one of her parents to fulfill the needs and functions she couldn't independently fulfill yet.

Shani was discharged after five months. She reached a minimum weight that she was allowed to maintain, and an outpatient treatment plan was established: psychotherapy and nutritional follow-ups. She moved to a small apartment where she lived on her own and was employed part-time in a job that kept her busy for several hours a day and added a small income. During the following years, this was an arrangement Shani consistently adhered to: she made it a point to work in a manner that wouldn't provide her with more than a small allowance. Over time it could be understood, in therapy, that this way she kept taking care of herself within her father's care; that this was one of the only ways she could feel that someone shares the burden with her.

At this initial point, a totally new situation was created, which was then strictly followed for several months. On the one hand, she'd undergone an immense change since prior to her hospitalization. She kept an apartment and a steady job, she followed her meal plan and she maintained her minimum weight. On the other hand, mentally she was still controlled by psychopathology: she was almost exclusively preoccupied with food and weight issues. In the mental functioning she was now establishing, the food and weight issues were her central selfobject components; being constantly engaged with them was the only way she knew how to "soothe" herself: false comfort, which fails to give peace, but at the same time cannot be let go of, fearing the familiar situation of total lack of protection.

The task in therapy was to build and reinforce the self, so that Shani would be able to protect herself from regressing back to her maladaptive functioning. The therapeutic work included the level of empathic relation and working through, on top of practical consideration of eating-disorder-related matters (in collaboration with the nutritional care). For example, Shani's anxiety of gaining weight was brought up in every session for months, with room given to expressing this anxiety. A lot of room was also given by the therapist to interpreting the origins of anxiety and associating those with letting go of control, of the uniqueness of thinness, and of the anorexic identity, which was the only thing Shani could hold on to. At the same time, a clear message was conveyed that she must gain weight notwithstanding this fear, namely, reach a physical condition that is not starvation. At one session when the scale showed a number higher than what she set for herself, she threw a temper tantrum and shouted at the therapist: "You betrayed me, you caused me to gain weight!", storming out of the room with the intention never to come back. She later regretted and said that she had nobody else she could trust. The therapist said that she gained weight by herself, but indeed it was encouraged by therapy and that she did not see this as betraying Shani but rather as protecting her. The therapist restated that she was convinced that by encouraging Shani to gain weight, she was protecting her and were she to give up this fight she would then betray her duty and Shani's best interest.

This message of the therapist's conviction that she was fighting for Shani's best interest, for Shani's healthy self and against destructive forces, was repeated countless times in therapy. It had to be repeated at different stages and contexts. First, there were many issues concerning the eating disorder. Shani had to learn how to make her meal plan more diverse and flexible, after she hadn't dared to slightly change any of its components, including meal hours, for a long time. She had to develop her ability to eat in public and change the nature of her physical exercise, which she forced herself to perform, from a tormenting activity to an enjoyable one. At the same time, her therapy touched upon areas that weren't related to food. At the beginning of therapy, all the dimensions of Shani's self-esteem were extremely low. Any reference, as minor as it may be, to an intellectual assignment or interpersonal communication immediately brought the response: "I am ugly and stupid, and it has no chance." Time and again she returned to the origin of these feelings: the way her mother looked at her; the way her father failed to look at her; her high school years that were spent in a spiral of diets, bingeing and purging. All she could think of in this period was the need to lose weight. She endlessly ruminated about what to eat, felt abandoned in her own home and unavailable for the conventional age-appropriate tasks. In the sessions, she could look back and see how no internal image of her academic or social abilities was ever established; these seemed like fields she could never succeed in.

The therapeutic work on these issues began already in the inpatient ward: the therapist attempted to capture any glimpse of a positive feeling of Shani toward herself, make room for it, highlight it and mirror it in a validating way. The psychological diagnosis process (through psychological testing) she had undergone at the ward provided the starting point. Some of its findings could be discussed in therapy, including highlighting the skills and abilities that were found. This gave an important initial foundation for her self-concept to develop, and she often used to return to this feedback throughout the following years in therapy.

This first glimpse was gradually augmented by additional experiences, and any such glimpse was fostered and reinforced in therapy. Upon her discharge from the hospital, Shani began to work toward completing her high school studies and worked on completing the missing matriculation exams. She then took the university's admission test, and to her surprise, she was accepted. All along this way, Shani's responses used to follow her existing patterns: she often returned to feelings of failure and tended to focus on difficulties rather than on success. In the therapy, she needed room to express these feelings and full acknowledgment of them. However, when such room was provided, she was sufficiently ready to thirstily absorb the consistent mirroring of her therapist that stressed her talents and successes. It seemed that apart from her natural skills, which enabled her to progress nicely throughout this long way, Shani had also had the ability to absorb all what she could gain from therapy. This allowed for more enthusiastic mirroring than she could ever gain exclusively by herself. The immense deficit was beginning to be filled, and Shani started to see herself as a person with skills, with a future and with a goal.

Another issue that had been present in therapy all along concerned the need of a validating selfobject. Throughout her illness, Shani had developed several ways to satisfy this need. Besides the endless pre-occupation with food, she was also preoccupied with occasional men with whom she was in love in her imagination. At the first stage, several men appeared in her immediate environment that took this role one after another and endlessly preoccupied her mind (at the hospital – one of the doctors; at school – one of the teachers; etc.). She would be preoccupied with a particular man and his whereabouts as if they were in a relationship ("today he was pissed off, I don't like it when he's angry," or "today he smiled, he is just adorable, it makes my day"). The therapist had a number of options: sometimes she chose to show Shani how she was using these thoughts and preoccupations, and at other times it appeared more important to provide emphatic mirroring for Shani's ability to feel enthusiasm and love. Shani accepted both levels, as if she had both levels in her simultaneously: falling in love played an important emotional role in her life, but she could also see the limits of an imaginary, unreal relationship. It seemed that she experienced the therapist's position as protecting her from letting herself believe that there was a real relationship, but only after the therapist acknowledged the significance of this experience, despite its realistic limitations.

The change in this field was the last to take place. The therapist realized that a new feeling was beginning to develop in Shani when, on the umpteenth time that such a narrative was repeated, her interventions were accepted differently. When the therapist attempted to show how this love existed only on Shani's mind, Shani was annoyed and argued that the therapist couldn't see that this time it was real. "This time a real relationship can truly develop." (The love object in question was a university professor, significantly older than her and married, who from Shani's stories seemed like a person surrounded with admiring students with no sign that he noticed Shani in particular.) This time, the therapist found it difficult to share Shani's delight and provide an empathic validation; rather, she stressed her understanding that such an impossible love was Shani's escape from possible relationships with her peers, who were starting to show their interest in her. Shani was angry at the therapist's refuse to share her experience and sensed the therapist's response as a failure to satisfy her narcissistic need of mirroring. But when she found out that the professor indeed did not respond to her suggestions, she was comforted by the feeling provided by the therapist's strength and understanding. Here, after experiencing the therapist's failure in providing validating mirroring, Shani could derive satisfaction of another narcissistic need, the need of an idealizable parent figure, through relying on the therapist's knowledge and understanding.

And indeed, the significant change emerged after this episode. The next time she talked about feeling excited and falling in love was with a guy her age, available and interested, for the first time of her life. Contrary to her imaginary love objects, this guy was as gentle as her; thus, the genuine relationship that was established here progressed very slowly. That way, for the first time, a relationship that is based on more mature self-selfobject relations could flower, with room for Shani's self, alongside her growing ability to see her partner as a distinct object, an autonomous source of initiative. This relationship with her boyfriend began to take form when the frequency of the therapy was reduced to two sessions a month, and Shani's reduced need of selfobject validation was apparent: one therapeutic hour every two weeks was enough to reinforce her confidence in the relationship's progress. As opposed to the panic she used to feel about interpreting any hint or working through any emotional fluctuation, in this relationship she already had the necessary self-strengths to digest and work through any new nuance of emotion and desire that sprouted in her.

Throughout therapy, Shani internalized the feeling that she is looked upon with eyes who believe in her ability to be healthy, to function normally and to enjoy regular things. It took a long time to establish her trust in therapy – both the psychotherapeutic and the nutritional – and inevitable empathic failures were part of building her strengths. Over time, the emphasis shifted to restoring Shani's faith in her ability to take care of herself, and in her ability to perceive herself as increasingly capable to hold herself, with a lower need to cling to figures who would serve as selfobjects for her.

This ability of Shani's self-holding was also developed through empathic failures. An example can be drawn from a later stage of the therapy. Shani already completed her undergraduate studies, she had a fuller social circle, she was working in a student job that contributed more substantially to her income and sessions had been taking place twice a month for a long time now. She had also been eating reasonably and maintained a steady weight for a long time. However, she wasn't completely free of her previous ideation, according to which she had to lose a little weight to be truly satisfied with herself. She therefore continued to meet the nutritionist every two weeks to measure her weight. In therapy, she occasionally assumed an obsessive preoccupation with the minor weight fluctuations, although practically it was quite obvious that since she eats regularly and maintained a steady weight, it is unreasonable to expect even a slight weight loss. The attempts to talk practically in therapy were rejected by Shani. It thus was gradually understood that Shani felt that were she to change anything of this ritual – the constant expectation to lose weight, the regular weighing and the futile meeting with the nutritionist – she would lose her anchor in the world. Checking with the nutritionist, it turned out that she, too, shared the therapist's feeling that Shani got addicted to the meal plan and the regular weighing and that it was necessary to help her to recover from this addiction. For a long time in therapy, the question was raised whether she wanted to change and free herself of this ritual element, and each time anew she rejected the idea. The therapist struggled with two optional directions: to accept her refusal to give up this anchor, perceiving it as a moderate version of the primary pathological core and continuing to explore this support with her; or to actively intervene in order to keep her from holding on to this ritual, even at the risk of Shani experiencing the therapist as un-empathic. For the time being, the therapist had no choice but to keep this internal struggle to herself.

One day, Shani returned to her obsessive preoccupation with her will to lose some weight, and even added some anger at the nutritionist for failing to cause her to lose weight. Furthermore, she said in a somewhat threatening tone "if it doesn't work, I'll go back to fasting and being anorexic." The therapist found herself reacting spontaneously, not out of an empathic exploration position, saying:

> Shani, whatever you do today this is your choice. You can choose to go back to eating patterns of fasting and anorexia, this is your life and your decisions. I am sorry I cannot convince you make the choice I find better: to stop expecting the nutritionist to fix your body and your weight, to stop even to set the goal of one kilogram more or less.

The therapist went on to say:

> You are in a healthy and stable weight, you can already trust your-
> self and your abilities, rather than continue and lean on weight
> measures and words of a nutritionist that for a long time now feels
> they are not necessary.

This was more of an emotional speech rather than a well-thought-of
therapeutic intervention, and Shani accepted it with resentment. She
left without really responding, only confirmed the next session in two
weeks. The therapist felt uncomfortable and somewhat concerned, ultimately phoned Shani and suggested to set an earlier date. Shani consented immediately, and when she arrived, she asked: "Are you tired
of treating me? When you said I could also choose going back to being
anorexic it seemed to me that you might be tired of me." Listening to
Shani, the therapist realized the heat of her response in the previous
meeting. She realized that when Shani "threatened" to go back to her
anorexic patterns, she, the therapist, felt anger at Shani for presenting a
state of regression as something desirable for her but threatening for the
therapist, as if Shani's own health was more of the therapist's concern
than Shani's. In the past, the therapist assumed this role of taking care
of Shani's self-functions when Shani wasn't capable of that. But the
anger she felt at Shani's threat showed her that at this point of therapy,
she does not feel it to be her role anymore. Today, she sees Shani as
someone capable of taking care of herself and this interaction made her
realize that Shani needed the push to do that. In the session, the therapist therefore discussed this understanding with Shani and explained
that she responded the way she did not because she was tired of Shani
but because she believed that Shani wouldn't go back to anorexic eating patterns. The therapist believes that Shani is too healthy for that.
Therefore, the therapist encourages her to let go of the weight measures,
the nutritionist and the meal plan and trusts her to continue her healthy
and stable condition by eating according to her own discretion. While
this message was already conveyed several times that way or another,
it was only now, following the empathic failure, that Shani could take
it in. A short while later, she indeed terminated the nutritional follow-
ups and began to try what she called "letting go." Besides discontinu-
ing the ritual of weighing and eating, she started to "let go" in other
areas as well. She approached a guy she was interested in, started to
attend social events that she previously feared and drew much delight
and excitement from these attempts.

Over time, Shani also achieved self-trust: her initial feeling of dependence on the therapist regarding working repeatedly through any thought and feeling has changed. Shani began to develop her own ability to calm herself down, to answer herself and believe in herself – and in turn, to love herself. Today, she looks healthy and happy. There is no trace of the thinness and anorexic morbidity at the time of admission.

It can be asked what was it that allowed Shani to go so far and so well. Can we estimate the therapy's role, compared to other factors in this success? Undoubtedly, Shani had a great ability to take advantage of therapy, to use the opportunity opened for her in order to recover from her eating disorder. It appears that even when she was deep into the disorder, she had buds of self that were seeking to grow. Her abilities to draw endless mirroring from her caretakers, and when this mirroring wasn't given to her – to learn and grow from empathic failures, to use her caretakers at any time and to see them as admirable figures – all suggest powers of self-growth that she had in her, and perhaps received early responsiveness and reinforcement. It is possible that although she did not reach in therapy memories of good parenting, such parenting in fact existed to a certain degree, as may be hinted by her father's helpful and appropriate involvement from when the disorder deteriorated, until this day. Such good parenting also allowed those buds to stay latent until they were provided with the nutrition necessary for their growth.

12 Searching for "Sweet Dreams" and the "Little Prince"

Yael Steinberg

This chapter will illustrate how food can substitute for a human selfobject in a case of a young woman with bulimia nervosa. The following case demonstrates how the development of an eating disorder and the changes that took place throughout therapy are connected to the loss of a close person. Food in this case serves as a dear friend, consoling and comforting, a loved one who is always present, unlike the close human beings who are experienced as hurting and disappointing.

Abby, a young woman in her early 20s, was referred to the inpatient ward at the hospital by a private therapist who saw Abby and her family. The suggestion to admit Abby to the hospital followed a deterioration in Abby's condition during the therapist's vacation, and Abby consented to be admitted. Before admission, Abby was experiencing several binges a day, which were accompanied by long rituals and ended in vomiting or in taking laxatives. Her weight dropped below the minimum weight and she ceased to menstruate.

Abby's eating disorder began several months after the death of her mother, who had suffered severe kidney failure for many years and undergone many hospital admissions. For years, the parents had concealed the mother's illness and its severity from Abby, who was the youngest daughter. Her older brother and sister were more involved and helped taking care of the mother.

Abby's preoccupation with dieting began upon leaving home for her army service and continued throughout the service. Toward Abby's discharge from the army, the mother's health further deteriorated. Simultaneously, Abby's preoccupation with diets has increased. Abby mother passed away a few months after Abby was discharged from the army. Several months later, Abby began to count calories and to significantly reduce the quantity of food she consumed, with occasional binges followed by vomiting or using laxatives. She managed to conceal her condition for quite some time.

At the time, Abby's brother studied and lived in an area remote from home, and her sister got married and moved to another town. Abby's father formed a new relationship with another woman and was often absent from home because of his work and the said relationship. As noted earlier, the beginning of Abby's deterioration was around the mother's death and the dissolution of the family unit. In fact, the seeds of the disorder can be traced back even earlier than leaving home for the army, and the disorder worsened after the completion of her military service.

Abby was hospitalized at the inpatient ward, and her professional team included a doctor, a psychologist, a nurse who was observing her closely and sat with her during meals and a nutritionist, who took care of adjusting the meal plan. In addition, family therapy sessions took place with the psychologist and a social worker.

In her first days in the hospital, Abby impressed the staff with her tidy appearance, her remarkable ability to pull herself together and the feeling she conveyed that she was here only for a focused, short-term therapy, and other than that she did not need the ward's services. Among those surrounding Abby, this image generated a special attitude and a willingness to approach her; but at the same time, they experienced her as distant and patronizing.

Abby was assigned a separate room in the psychiatric ward, to which she brought many personal belongings that created a home-like look. The way she arranged the room probably suggested her need of a home, of a warm and soft touch; yet it also made a statement of her self-sufficiency and her ability to take care of herself without needing or depending on others.

The special attitude toward Abby and the wish to get closer to her on the one hand, and the sense of distance on the other hand, were also apparent in our relationship. Abby aroused my curiosity. She struck me as an intelligent young woman, her voluntary admission attested to her motivation for therapy and the sense of great vulnerability beyond her appearance made me want to take care of her. However, my attempts to get to know her beyond her presented symptoms were quickly met by resistance, and I sensed that Abby remained cold and distant. She made it clear to me that she didn't want to gain weight but simply get rid of her endless thoughts about food. Other than that, she didn't think that she had any problem, and she didn't think she was too thin. She enjoyed her physical appearance and the attention it earned her.

Abby always showed up on time for sessions, wearing soft sweatpants that usually serve to wear at home, and she cuddled herself on the couch in a way that resembled a TV couch. Usually she started by asking how

I was or making a comment about items or pictures in the therapists' room. Sometimes she organized items that were dislocated or expressed concern for dehydrated plants. On the one hand, this approach attested to Abby's ability to take care of others and feel concern for them. On the other hand, it also entailed something characteristic of concern for a room at home, a wish to make the room familiar and comfortable, a place where one can receive therapy and grow.

The contents brought up in the sessions typically concerned the daily life at the ward: the meals, the pain of meeting the meal plan's demands and the limitation imposed on Abby as part of the hospitalization program. I attempted to relate to the contents she brought up, to stay as close as possible to her experience, without interpretations or attempts to link her past with the here and now. This position had been consolidated after attempts to offer such interpretations, even if appeared to me very right, remained considerably distant from her, failed to touch her and maybe even reduced or shut her down. For instance, she brought up her difficulty about eating certain items of the meal plan, her feeling that she was being overfed without anyone responding to her requests, or the difficulty to go through the "boring" evening time when there are fewer staff members and there is hardly any activity in the ward. Abby talks about boredom and I say that the boredom increases when the staff members leave and she is left alone. I choose to leave out the connection to her feeling when she was left alone after her mother died and the home was dissolved. Despite Abby's request to get rid of her annoying thoughts about food and of the accompanying behavior, I make it clear that before we get rid of those, perhaps it is better to understand what they are telling us.

Symptom-wise, the binges, the vomiting and the use of laxatives all terminated upon Abby's admission to the ward. All in all, Abby manages quite well to meet the demands of meals, which she eats while being accompanied by the nurse assigned to her.

Therapy and the ward in general serve as some sort of a warm home, organized (with five meals a day), with extended "family" (the staff and the rest of the patients) in which Abby feels understood. It appears that the feeling of holding they provide reduces the sense of threat and reinforces her sense of control. From this position, where she feels safer, she begins to increasingly trust other people, and her external image – of a self-sufficient person capable of taking care of herself, who does not need the ward but for a brief treatment – is gradually softening.

Abby begins to be in touch with her feelings and share them with me; she is able, through her experience of hospitalization, to recall her mother's countless hospitalizations and cry out of agony, pain and guilt.

The turning point that signaled a new phase in treatment was the first bingeing and vomiting that took place while in treatment. This event, occurring within the ward, paved the road for better understanding the connection of bingeing and purging to the relationships with people. Abby first throws up in the ward after the staff decides not to let her go out two days before a party celebrating her father's promotion. The decision was made after it turned out in therapy that Abby means to use these two days to prepare the menu and the food for the party. The underlying rationale was that letting Abby organize the food for the party means putting her in an almost impossible position, thereby collaborating with her façade of taking care of other people's needs without attending to her illness and her need to be taken care of.

This decision of the staff stirs a difficult feeling in me that I betrayed Abby, that I let her down and now I would probably lose her because she wouldn't trust me or want to share anything with me ever again.

Indeed, in the following session Abby is silent all through the hour. I try to find out how she feels, but it's like she is standing behind a wall of glass, and the silence in the room is thick and irritating. The same night, Abby eats anything she had at her possession, and vomits it all, but later tells the nurse what she did. The nurse, understanding this as a reaction for the staff's decision, suggests that Abby talks about it in therapy. The next session, Abby shows up seemingly calm, and during the conversation she recalls the nurse's suggestion to talk about the incident. In the conversation, she can tell me she is mad at me for betraying her, but her affect does not convey anger. I find it hard to relate to the anger directed at me, and try to show her how her anger is translated to an action of bingeing and purging, following which her anger is calmed down, and the bad feeling of the previous session disappears.

I also understand that if it wasn't for the nurse's suggestion to talk with me about the incident, there would probably be no traces of the disappointment and anger or of the bingeing and purging. In other words, without the containment offered by the nurse, who helped Abby to preserve and contain the incident, the disappointment and anger would have probably been mitigated and forgotten like the food that disappeared without a trace.

But what I could only later understand was that as far as Abby was concerned, by preventing her from preparing the party for her father, we put her in a position of letting her father and her family down, and letting them down meant losing them, just as I felt that if I let her down I would lose her. The emerging disappointment and anger are so dangerous and problematic that both Abby and I find our ways to avoid them; I evade them within the conversation, and she turns to food.

Another binge followed by taking laxatives that took place around a holiday home visit further clarifies the connection between disappointment by someone and the binge. Abby is given a special permission to go to a holiday dinner at the home of her relatives. She plans to go home first, meet her brother and then go to the dinner with him. Abby is thrilled about the event and tells me she loves family dinners and the atmosphere.

Abby leaves the ward early to be on time. She arrives home, gets ready and waits for her brother, who was supposed to arrive at four o'clock. Fifteen minutes before four o'clock he calls and says he'd be a little late. Abby turns to the refrigerator and eats some things but makes a real effort not to eat anything she knows that would make her want to vomit. After an hour, he calls again saying he got stuck at a friend's house on his way, and further delay is expected. Abby finds it hard to hold on. Her brother eventually arrives at eight, after Abby already devoured, gradually, the entire contents of the refrigerator and took laxatives. When her brother finally arrives, she urges him to go to the family dinner by himself, lying to him that she already had plans with her boyfriend. In her conversation with me the next day, there is no sign of her previous day's expectation or disappointment. Abby relates the event indifferently, saying she is used to it, that in fact she expected nothing else. I feel how my gut is twisting in anger at Abby's brother. I try to "digest" for her, to hold and to return her some of my gut feelings; feelings that, meanwhile, she has managed to empty and lose. I also remind her of yesterday's expectation and show her how she turns to food like a comforting friend who is always there to soothe and console her when she is hurt and disappointed. I showed her how things turn upside down; rather than seeing her brother as hurting and disappointing, rather than being angry at him, she becomes the one who is hurting others with her lies and disappointing with her behavior, and ultimately, she is angry at herself.

The gap between the intensity of my own emotional response and Abby's emotional detachment is particularly striking concerning those events. It seems that Abby deposited with me her unbearable intensity of anger and of fear to disappoint and to lose. It feels that she conveys her feelings from gut to gut, which is probably what makes me hurry to the dining room after my conversations with her.

The end of Abby's hospitalization is approaching, and she earns more home leaves. She also starts to vomit more, but she can see me and talk with me about the connection of her bulimic behavior to her disappointment of someone she thought she could trust. She talks a lot about the "little prince" (a kind of ice cream) and "sweet dreams" (a kind of chocolate bar), which she can look for anywhere, and I can talk with her about the guaranteed and tangible pleasure that "sweet dreams" and "little prince" provide, versus the disappointment and uncertainty that emerge in her encounter with reality and with her close ones.

It seems that the connection Abby discovers between her emotions and behaviors sparks her curiosity about herself and her relations with others. Her ability to touch what underlies the binges and the purging behaviors, and the attempt to understand it, reinforces Abby's feeling that I understand her and that she understands herself. The attempt to achieve understanding provides her with a new tool for coping and control, and she's trying to use it. The feeling of understanding and being understood also allows her to be more open without the need to conceal things from me.

The shift from full hospitalization in the inpatient ward to halfway-out framework was accompanied by an abrupt change of symptoms. Immediately upon the shift, daily binges emerged, sometimes occurring even more than once a day. In one of the sessions before her discharge, Abby shows up with a long list of questions regarding the future of our therapy, reflecting her anxiety of the change and her fear of being abandoned. Among other questions, Abby asks if it is possible to be hospitalized again. I mirror her anxiety of leaving the ward, but nonetheless I am also frightened and anxious about the deterioration of her symptoms. Like Abby, I also feel alone without the team's protection and support, and I feel that the minute she walks out of the session and goes home, I lose control.

At the same time, it seems that understanding and interpreting the behavior do not suffice to comfort Abby and that she needs a more holding environment. Consequently, I recruit the team again and together we set up a clearer and stricter framework shared by additional team members. Likewise, the team makes it clear to Abby that continuing the deterioration would lead to readmission in the ward. These actions appear to help her gain better control over the binges. She says that she controls them better because of her fear of a second hospitalization, but it also appears that what was presented to her as a threat was perceived by her as a promise that we wouldn't leave her, a promise she could come back; thus it also served to comfort her.

The dramatic change surrounding leaving the ward makes it clear to me how much the staff and the ward, beyond our individual therapy, satisfied Abby's need of a framework providing basic safety and vitality, a need that was completely undermined when her home was emptied and disintegrated.

In fact, her hospitalization brought all family members together for the family therapy, a reunion that seldom happened before. Namely, through her illness and hospitalization Abby also managed to "hold" her family together.

In the next several months, the therapy took place in the outpatient clinic. The most apparent theme in the sessions of this period is the connection Abby discovers between feelings of loneliness, emptiness and boredom and her bulimic behavior.

Within the sessions, there is a feeling of warmth and closeness. During the sessions, Abby explores her relationships with people around her, family, boyfriends, female friends and the feelings aroused surrounding these relationships. Our conversations become richer, both in terms of contents and in terms of affect, which together create a feeling of vitality. The preoccupation with very tangible things and the feelings of coldness and reduction characteristic of the talks at the beginning of therapy almost disappeared.

In Abby's relationship with me, a wish for closeness and dependence is emerging. Abby tells me about a dream in which she comes to visit me and plays with my children. Before a holiday, she calls me to wish me happy holidays and tells me about a significant experience with her boyfriend. I feel she tells me about her boyfriend and about what happened to her like a daughter sharing with her mother.

Along the sessions, she slowly discovers how her hunger is aroused in specific times and places. Apparently, she only binges when she is home alone. In one of the most touching conversations of this period, she tells me about a feeling of coldness, emptiness and alienation at home. She has an intense feeling of emptiness because since her mother's death almost nobody lives there apart from Abby. She can see how the sensation of hunger that she feels when she is home alone disappears at others' homes, like at her sister's home or her boyfriend's home; there it feels like family with the liveliness of people coming and going. It seems like the binge that occurs when she is alone has two sides: on the one hand, it is obvious that she feels empty, lonely and bored when she is home alone; on the other hand, she relates her need to avoid those surrounding her or to push them away in order to allow herself to enjoy the binge, what occasionally sounds like a secret rendezvous with a lover or with the "little prince." It seems that she would make any effort to find a supermarket or a convenience store open, even in the middle of the night, to find "sweet dreams" or a package of the "little prince," instead of risking sweet dreams or waiting for her prince.

Later on, Abby better manages to link hunger to relationships in which she feels important and understood. She notices how her hunger disappears when she is with her boyfriend, and he is available and relates to her. She can also say at the beginning of a session that she is willing to binge this very minute, but later on, after a moment of closeness between us in which she feels understood, she says the hunger is gone for now, although she knows it would come back the moment she leaves the room. She tells me how much she enjoys family gatherings, delighted with the family atmosphere, the joy, the togetherness, and she discovers that although food is accessible in such events, she feels no need to binge.

Turning to food as a substitute for someone who can satisfy and comfort her is raised independently regarding a vacation Abby takes with her boyfriend out of town. They take a vacation with two other couples of friends, and one evening they all go out together and Abby feels neglected by her boyfriend. She looks at the other couples and feels very lonely and hurt. When they return to the hotel, Abby feels an intense need to go out to buy some food and eat it, but she restrains herself, and instead of bingeing she sits down and writes me a letter. In the letter, she details the situation and discloses the feeling that she has no one in the world who truly loves her, and how badly she wanted to go out that moment and buy herself as much "sweet dreams" as she pleases and eat them because for her, food is the only thing that really exists. Through that letter, I could realize that Abby was beginning to see me as someone who exists for her also between sessions, and she tries to cling on to me and use me as a substitute for food rather than the other way around.

The last stage of therapy begins with my announcement on my forthcoming leaving. In parallel to the termination of therapy, Abby's father was supposed to go overseas for several weeks for business, and her sister was supposed to deliver her baby. All these events intensely raise the threat of separation. Abby's response is a sharp increase in the frequency of bingeing and purging, up to more than once a day at the point of termination. This reaction resembles the deterioration around the separation from the previous therapist (which led to her hospital admission), and around the separation from the ward, but this time Abby is more capable to relate to her feelings. She talks about her sense of emptiness and feeling that nobody really cares for her; her sister is busy with her pregnancy and upcoming delivery, her father – with his work, and I am leaving, too. She shows up to one session looking pale, tired, apathetic and distant. When I try to find out what's happening, she tells me she vomited before coming in, and I feel how emptiness can become so tangible. Emptiness is evident in her appearance, her affect and her themes in therapy. The feelings of closeness, warmth and vitality that began to surface now fade away.

In one session, Abby talks about her relationship with her sister and of her pregnancy. She describes how her sister is growing fatter, and I see how Abby is diminishing. She talks about her wish to get married and to be a mother, a mother who is needed and necessary. When I ask how she would feel if she gains weight during pregnancy, she says that by then she wouldn't mind because she would have a family of her own, a husband and a child, so it wouldn't matter how she'd look. It seems that against the dreadful emptiness, accompanied by feeling of nonexistence, Abby tries to be filled, but to no avail. However, wishes to be filled with something else start to emerge, something alive that would give her a sense of worth, that would need her and wouldn't separate from her.

Around the deterioration of Abby's condition, it is very difficult for me to leave her and I try hard to find a suitable facility for her. Her father also decides to defer his business trip. Once again, I feel the illness's power to "hold together."

Abby and I terminate our therapy, but she continues therapy in a new framework in which she holds on and establishes a good relationship. It seems that therapy helped her to believe anew in the option of getting help from someone else. After another two years of therapy, she made a considerable improvement that enabled her to let go of the severe symptoms she was initially admitted with.

13 Patients With Eating Disorders and Latent Idealization Needs

Sara Haramati

Self psychology views the idealizing need as an important developmental need: this is one of the poles of the self's structure as we saw in Chapter 2. For healthy development to take place, the self must experience validation, mirroring and acknowledgment by a selfobject, as well as idealization toward this selfobject. Kohut discussed the self's basic need to merge with what is experienced as the selfobject's strength and stability (Kohut, 1971; Wolf, 1995).

Throughout normal development, any idealized parental figure would manifest disappointing aspects. Minor, digestible disappointments typically occur gradually and in a manner that allows to work through the undermining of that idealization. This working through leads to internalization of parental functions and development of self-functioning. In normal development, this process also depends on the self-functioning of the parent: his or her self-esteem, the ability to allow admiration directed at them and the ability to contain the disappointment directed at them.

Patients bring to therapy their need of an idealizable figure. According to self psychology, the therapist must let the idealization process happen, despite the difficulties it poses for most therapists. Kohut's seminars (Kohut, 1987b) offer an illustration of his approach to this issue. Kohut responds to a description of a therapist who dismissed the patient's thanks and emphasizes that it is important not to interfere with the patient's need to have idealizable therapists. If the value of gratitude is properly acknowledged, it can play a significant role in achieving normal mental structure. In that case, the patient achieved better self-acceptance and cohesiveness when she related to an accepting and idealizable figure – the therapist.

Accepting the patient's idealization contributes to strengthening her self-structure. Nevertheless, it is not always easy for the therapist to allow it. Kohut (1968) explains that the difficulty in accepting the patient's idealization occurs when the *therapist's* grandiose self is not properly analyzed; in this state of affairs, idealization directed at the therapist would stimulate unconscious grandiose fantasies and lead to reinforcing the defense mechanisms thereof. This would lead the therapist to reject the patient's idealizing transference.

Sands (1989), too, talks about the need to allow the patient to fully express her idealization needs. She warns of rejecting the idealization because of the therapists' discomfort about it and the grandiosity it evokes in them as well as of interpreting the idealization as defense against hostility.

The difficulty of appropriately treating the patient's idealization needs is even more substantial in the cases I present next. In these cases, the idealization needs are often latent. The patients do not treat the therapist with admiration but tend to be hostile and critical. I suggest that this very behavior reflects unsatisfied idealization needs.

The patients I wish to describe tend to convey conflicting messages: they typically express desperate wish to satisfy very basic needs and at the same time act to destroy any opportunity for these needs to be satisfied. It is often the case that an understanding and empathic approach on the part of the therapist might insatiably provoke and stimulate the need for acceptance. Empathic mirroring and interpretations then lead to escalation of frustration and anger toward the therapist, self-destruction behaviors or both, a process well-described by Slochower (1991). Newman (1980) and Bachar (2000) describe defense against the need for understanding and empathy and its concealment in patients whose need was frustrated in childhood. I suggest that, similarly, where the idealization need was severely frustrated in childhood, we would witness defense and concealment of this need. The challenging behaviors of such patients can thus be seen as latently expressing their idealization needs.

I therefore propose a therapeutic stance that might be effective and beneficent for these patients: a therapeutic stance that enables the patient to experience idealization toward the therapist and thus meets these latent needs. Through this stance, the therapist provides the patient with the following message:

> I hear your needs, I understand the pain and frustration you feel when these needs are frustrated. I hear the frustration you feel towards *me* when I fail to satisfy your needs the way you need me to. At the same time, I feel that I am a good therapist for you.

This is a message demonstrating the therapist's faith and confidence in her ability to absorb idealization even in the face of devaluative messages on the patient's part. The following vignettes illustrate this concept.

Tania is a 20-year-old student, suffering from eating disorders since her early adolescence. She is the second of three children. Her father, a strict and demanding man, is a CEO of a high-tech company, and her mother, a secretary, is a bitter and frustrated woman. Throughout her entire child-hood, Tania experienced them as judgmental and felt they never accepted her for who she was. At 15, Tania manifested prodromal anorexia, which was halted thanks to a focused therapeutic intervention. But Tania remained extremely preoccupied with eating and dieting, an obsession that caused her great pain. This was the motivation to contact me for therapy.

Through the intake sessions, Tania expressed considerable hostility and disappointment. It was my impression that she expected me to offer an immediate cure the minute she briefly presents the problem to me. She responded impatiently to my questions about her background, to my interest in her thoughts and feelings and to my explorative attempts. I tried to explain the nature of therapy and to offer a therapeutic plan. But I was hardly surprised at the end of the intake sessions when Tania announced that she could not commence therapy because of a training program she was undertaking. I experienced her as angry and disap-pointed with the entire process.

For that reason, I was surprised when Tania contacted me two months later telling me that now she could begin therapy. I was all the more surprised of the good use to which she put the sessions: she talked about her relationships with her mother and a friend of hers, about her doubts and her reflections. She responded more acceptingly to my interven-tions and seemed as if she could enjoy my validating mirroring. I thus found myself completely unprepared when around the tenth session, she suddenly asked whether there was a point for her to continue therapy, since it didn't seem to help her. I tried to inquire about this feeling of hers and to get to the bottom of the gap between our perceptions. Tania rejected all my attempts and argued that the therapy meant nothing for her. I noticed, however, that when I agreed to terminate, Tania seemed deeply disappointed by my consent. At that point, I was too exhausted to see that she sought my own faith in the therapy.

It took me a while to see this. Tania returned to therapy a while after this break. Variations of this theme were repeated occasionally along the years of therapy: Tania's complaints about me and disappointment of me at unexpected points, which left me frustrated and helpless. How-ever, I slowly realized that what she yearned for at these points more than anything was my own confidence in the therapeutic process and my ability to help her.

Over time, I had elaborated the therapeutic stance I found suitable for those times, when Tania harshly conveyed her feeling that I wasn't able to help her. Instead of surrendering to exhaustion and burnout, I chose to reply: "Tania, I am helping you. This is my ability to make an effect – I can't completely stop your suffering, although I wish I could. I can talk with you, be with you and understand you."

Julia, 18 years old, had suffered from eating disorders since age 16. She comes from a family with multiple problems. Her father was unemployed for years and "supported" his family by pressing the local municipality and the social services. Her mother had never been employed, and it appeared that she was using her six children for her own needs, by keeping them close to her. Julia, the third child, learned her father's patterns of demands and threats as a way to fulfill her needs. When she developed her eating disorder, she used to make threats of self-harm to have her needs fulfilled.

In our eating disorders unit, Julia seemed to need constant attention and responsiveness and tended to complain about the staff and the therapists whenever she felt they were failing to meet these needs. When she felt disappointed or frustrated, she used to react by dramatic demonstration of her difficulty to eat.

The first therapeutic step was an attempt to understand Julia's tendency to threaten to harm herself. The therapy was based on empathic understanding and interpretation of the destructive behavior as expressing genuine, unfulfilled needs. This therapeutic stance evoked in Julia an insatiable hunger for more and more of this understanding attitude. What she could do to get more of that was escalate and deteriorate her disordered behavior. Even after we understood that we must set some boundaries, we failed to do so effectively.

The turning point occurred once we altered this therapeutic stance. The change stemmed from understanding Julia's behavior as expressing her longing for an idealizable caretaking figure: a figure possessing confidence and faith of his or her therapeutic ability, who would be able to provide both empathic understanding of her needs and boundaries for her destructive behaviors, in a confidently beneficent manner.

Now I started to respond differently whenever Julia entered the cycle of devaluation and deprecation of me, supplemented with threats to lose weight and hurt herself. Whenever she did that, I told her I hoped she could control her destructive impulse because if she actualized her threats, it would terminate her treatment plan at our unit. I told her I believed it was important for her to stay in our care because I saw how helpful it was for her. Each time, I described at length why I thought our program was good for her – because it took care of her genuine and painful needs. Julia really loved that part: her eyes were gleaming and she could hardly hide her smile when I spoke. After these talks, Julia looked calmer and more pleasant.

Now Julia seemed hungry for this more confident and idealizable approach more than for the previous approach. It seemed to me that she was waiting to conclude any therapeutic interaction with my speech of the importance of our program for her. I felt how rare and meaningful it was for her that a caretaking figure would be strong and confident and accept her idealization.

In these cases, acknowledging the patients' need of my own faith and confidence in my ability as a therapist was a turning point in therapy. Both women had no ability in the beginning of the process to handle increasing stress or need: in the sessions, intensification of the need without its immediate fulfillment brought about anger and frustration toward the therapist. Outside the sessions, the frustrated need led to anger manifestation toward the self through disordered eating behaviors and self-harm. When I perceived this recurring pattern as an expression of idealization needs, I was provided with a new therapeutic stance: a position of articulating my confidence in my ability.

Expressing such confidence, even if felt by the therapist, is uncomfortable. As therapists, we are used to constantly scrutinizing and criticizing ourselves. But Julia and Tania made me realize how much they needed a therapist figure who is confident in her care's adequacy and can survive their devaluation and deprecation.

Tania's therapy is now on its third year; she now has a more cohesive self. She describes her ability to comfort herself from time to time when her stress or anxiety increases and her ability to hold back until she calms down. She tells me that she already has strength to cope with her immense hunger for unconditional acceptance and understanding, for love, for attention and for food as well! Today she can tell me that she fondly remembers the times when I knew what she needed and I was confident in my ability to help her, and how much this time gave her strength.

This illustrates a new manifestation of idealization needs, different than the more familiar theme of the patient idealizing the therapist and the therapist who moves uneasily in the chair in the face of such admiration. Here I want to suggest that the patient attempts to convey her wish to idealize the therapist in a negative and paradoxical manner.

As far as such patients are concerned, the need of an idealizable figure is an unsatisfied need. It can originate in disappointment at the parent who was not able to be idealized, disappointment bigger than the ability to work it through. When it happens, it can lead to denial of self needs (Kohut, 1971, 1977b). This developmental deficit is often evident in patients with eating disorders: disappointment of the primary environment's ability to provide comfort and containment sometimes leads to the use of food as substitute for the ideal selfobject (Sands, 1989).

Recognizing such a flaw in the idealization process may lead to recognize the patient's idealization needs even when they are expressed in negative and paradoxical terms. The devaluing manifestation is typically a very unsettling event for the therapist, often leading to doubts as to his or her understanding and abilities. Epstein (1987), Slochower (1991) and other scholars describe countertransference responses evoked by these "challenging" patients – feelings of anger, destructiveness and insecurity.

It is my contention here that the therapist's ability to maintain a sense of self-worth in such cases and accept the idealization allows for reparation and development of self-functions. I will conclude with Kohut's words in one such case:

> In the transference his fear was not, as I had erroneously believed for a while, that he could never match my achievements but, on the contrary, that I would knuckle under when belittled and attacked . . . he wanted me not to hide my strengths and achievements but to display them proudly and openly.
>
> (Kohut, 1984, p. 151)

14 Absolute Autonomy

Myrna Milun

Lara was 22 when she arrived at the eating disorders clinic. An assured, stylish and attractive young woman, intelligent and well-spoken with an engaging smile, she immediately declared herself an adherent of "absolute autonomy." She believed in independence in all spheres of life and was determined to conduct herself without help or interference from others. She was adamant that her parents were not responsible for her condition; she alone was to blame. Her bulimia was not due to psychological causes but rather to habit. She did not think that there was much chance of a cure but was aware that things had gotten out of control. This was the first time she had decided on her own to turn to therapy. In the past, her parents had sent her as a result of their anxiety about her weight.

Lara grew up in a small town. Her parents were educated and hardworking. She was the middle child of three siblings. From the age of ten, she experienced herself as overweight and received hints from her family that they felt she ate too much. Unhappy with her appearance, she tried to restrict her eating. She was successful in her studies but not in the social realm and frequently stayed home from school, claiming stomach pains. She lost weight gradually until she reached 36 kg without her family noticing the severity of her condition. The restrictive behavior became very difficult for her and the anorexia developed into bulimia. The symptoms appeared only at home. She felt that her disorder did not affect her life outside of home. Three years later, her mother heard her purging and referred her to a therapist.

In high school, her social life improved and she became active in a youth movement. After graduation, she left therapy. Frequently alone at home, she ate "forbidden foods." She gradually gained weight. She began to dance and joined a dance troupe, started university studies and moved out of home. Lara made a conscious decision to leave the bulimia at her parents' home, to keep her new home, her autonomous space, "clean." She did not prepare cooked meals and lost weight. Her mother sent her to therapy again. A relationship with a young man developed. Despite some difficulties, she felt the relationship was "healing" and supportive. When they separated after a few months, a year before she began therapy with me, she purged in her apartment for the first time. From then on, she was not able to limit the symptoms to her parents' home, a situation which became increasingly distressful to her.

Lara declared that she felt alone, unable to regulate or contain herself. That was what brought her to therapy. She was very busy studying and working during the week. On weekends, she returned to the family home. There, without her normal busy schedule, she was overcome by a feeling of emptiness, in response to which she binged and purged. She was aware that the symptoms were triggered by feelings of loneliness and boredom. When she was active, she felt that the food went to the right places; when she was inactive, there was no justification in her mind for the amount of food she ate. She had not earned the right to eat. She felt bored, empty, scared and threatened. The bingeing connected her with her body, a kind of grounding. She felt the binge was a place of regression that she preserved and could not renounce. At this time in the therapy, Lara clung to her ideal view of her family as providing a safe haven, a place where there was room for her, where she was fully accepted. Despite this, she did not feel calm at her parents' home. I surmised that all was not as safe and secure as it seemed and that Lara was using the bingeing as a way of dealing with complicated feelings she could not express directly.

She did not like to bother others, to ask for help, to complain. She did not feel comfortable expressing her needs openly and did not like to criticize others or argue. At home or away, she always maintained a façade of well-being. Her parents bought into this pretense too easily. She was the good child who did not have special needs or demand attention as her siblings did. On the other hand, she described a concerted effort to suit herself to the needs of others, especially in her dancing, where she needed to simultaneously be aware of herself, her body, her own place, while considering that of her partner, the intentions of the choreographer and the response of the audience. It was a struggle for her to insert her needs into the system, being so attuned to the needs of the other. The intricate "dance" with the other demanded a great deal of her. Nothing was ever simple, nothing ever perfect. She was always self-conscious, never satisfied, could never rest on her laurels. She was never gratified by praise, always wanting more. She felt it was built into the nature of professional dancing.

I began to see the area of the symptoms as her private realm, her autonomy, her place where she could do as she pleased, not suit herself to others, a place where she could make her own "mess." This was her safe haven, where she could make place for her needs. She described in more detail what happened at home when she was in her bulimic state. Before the beginning of the family meal, she enters into a state of madness, a bubble, alienated from everyone else present, occupied with taking food, eating and purging. Her family watch with trepidation but have learned from experience not to interfere. She is alone in her private world, with herself, her body, in the most concrete sense. The binge soothes her more than being with her family does despite the fact that they love and accept her.

In my understanding, Lara needed a way to soothe herself from the distress of not being seen enough by others, a way to manage the hurt and maintain her feelings of self-worth in the absence of sufficient acknowledgment from others. The binge and subsequent purge served as concrete compensation for the lack of narcissistic "food," emotional confirmation from others, human selfobject functions. For this reason, it was so difficult to give up on this space, which could not find expression elsewhere. The Lara who binges and purges is split off from the Lara who pleases and who does not bother others. In this private space, Lara is more impulsive, spontaneous, and maybe not even really nice. At this stage, Lara did not identify with my thoughts on the matter.

I became more and more aware, during the first months of the therapy, that I was making a special effort to listen to Lara. She impressed me with her knowledge of art and culture, and I found myself anxious not to have my ignorance exposed. I tried to keep up with her verbal fluency and speed, the intellectual content of her speech, trying to understand everything she said. I became aware that she was making me feel what she herself felt, the need to work hard at the complicated "dance" with the other, to suit myself to her. Together with this, I also felt that she distanced me with her intellectualizations, that she found difficulty in allowing me to be experienced as close, in allowing herself to become dependent on my empathic responses. She needed to protect her autonomous space and allowed me only a limited glimpse into her private world.

In time, however, some chinks appeared in her armor. A close family member became ill and Lara participated in his care. This involved family interaction that was not focused around meals as on the weekend or festivals. The sense of togetherness in this endeavor was positive and fulfilling. Lara felt that her contribution was meaningful and recognized by the family. In addition, she appeared in a public appearance that was highly praised, and this pleased her. This was the first time she acknowledged the beneficial effect on her of being applauded. Lara reported eating and feeling satisfied, a rare occurrence. There had been no binges for some time. She had not felt the need to resort to food to compensate for unbearable feelings of emptiness. She was more emotionally satisfied, enjoying the positive effects on her feelings of self-worth from rewarding human interaction. I said that the positive experience of being acknowledged was fulfilling and that she did not need to fill herself with food. She was able to remain on the emotional track and not to cross over to the food track. Lara was beginning to understand the emotional underpinnings of her "habit" as she had called her disorder. However, she was still afraid to be dependent on others for her emotional well-being. She wanted to break the habit of bingeing and purging but still found it difficult to struggle against the urge to do so.

After four months in therapy, Lara reported a general improvement, feeling calmer, having fewer binges. She found she could begin to fight the urge. She occasionally referred to the therapy as beneficial but never directly referred to me. I understood that she could not recognize me as having any direct impact on her feelings or behavior. She was able to say that she was not convinced my understanding was accurate and that it was too simplistic or "psychological," but she never expressed hurt or anger. She said that it was difficult for her to accept an explanation that came from without, from another place, but that she was also aware that when previous therapists had just gone along with her, nothing happened, nothing changed. I said that I understood the importance of hearing her and remaining close to her experience but that she also needed me to help her integrate the different parts of herself that she felt were not connected. This felt right to her.

She completed her studies and was involved in many performances and had to cancel sessions. After a month's break, she reported losing the momentum and finding difficulty in fighting the urge to binge. She planned to move to another city with a more vibrant cultural life that would afford her the chance to find more work opportunities and possibly a meaningful relationship, which had eluded her for some time. Her plans had not yet taken shape and she felt insecure and not grounded. She binged but found it to be an unwelcome experience and was happy that bingeing was losing its power over her.

I was surprised to receive an invitation from her to attend a performance of hers. She felt I could understand her more deeply if I saw her in action. I was excited to be invited to enter more intimately into her personal space. I was truly impressed by the quality of her performance. Lara could not see that I was in the audience but was happy that I came. She felt good about her performance, but when she saw photographs of it, she felt overweight and gave in to the urge to binge and purge again.

She was working on an independent project, spending much time alone and bingeing more.

Lara could not look at herself in the mirror, hated what she saw there and was not satisfied with her body. She found it hard to like herself. She said her parents valued efficiency and productivity, without dispensing much admiration. This was the first time she alluded to any lack of empathy from home, the first time I felt she acknowledged any empathic insight from me about the emotional atmosphere at home. She was well aware of the long road ahead to internalization of the feeling of self-acceptance and self-love.

During the holiday season, she was at home for an extended period. She was irritable and angry without understanding why, bingeing and purging every day. On investigation, it appeared that there was a new baby in the family who had been the center of attention. Lara had not been able to bring herself and what was important to her to the attention of the family. She was frustrated, agitated and felt unregulated. I suggested that the baby had stolen all the limelight, that there had not been enough place for her. She escaped to the familiar autonomous space of symptoms. For the first time, my understanding resonated with her. She desired to distance herself somewhat from the family where she felt too little acknowledgment. They had always been "nice." There had never been room for rebellion. She had not managed in the context of the family to define herself or her special place. In the past, she had always been careful not to take up too much room at the expense of the others, not to burden them with her issues. I said that was why she went off to her space, the pathological one, the place where she did not pander to the others' needs. Then she filled herself up, was disgusted with herself for taking too much for herself, for giving room to her needs and had to purge. With this understanding, she managed not to binge and purge over the weekend. She had managed to regulate herself.

Lara searched for integration between the different parts of her identity, the city girl, the small-town girl, the artist, the nonconformist, the good girl. She said that there were parts of her that were more true and authentic, and parts that were more false, aimed at pleasing others. In her creative endeavors, she tried to express herself and not merely please and impress the audience. She endeavored to find her place. She managed in her dancing more than in the interpersonal sphere. She still found it difficult to regulate her eating, to establish the accurate amount to eat. She understood that her difficulty in regulating her eating was connected to her difficulty in regulating her emotions. Her growing insight into this connection helped her to reduce her bingeing and purging again by focusing more on attempting to achieve emotional regulation in a more direct way.

Lara met a young man, also an artist, who saw her dance and was attracted to her. She was enthusiastic, found the relationship exciting, emotional and intense. She seemed to glow from within. She was able to ease up on food as never before. She ate well with her boyfriend, was less rigid, more adventurous in her eating. She made it clear that the flag of the autonomous space was still flying, however, and that she did not agree to become dependent on someone else in order to rid herself of symptoms, to admit to needing someone else. I remarked on how difficult it was for her to allow herself to be on the receiving end in the relationship. I said that it was important to have support and empathy but also acknowledged her need to feel that her inner core was becoming stronger, more cohesive.

The relationship deepened. Lara shared with me details of their growing intimacy and the delicate "dance" in the search for the accurate distance between them. She feared losing herself in the relationship and was determined to maintain her social and professional endeavors so as not to be entirely taken up with her boyfriend. I reflected that she felt more self-confident, that there was an emergence of the sparks of a developing inner self, but I also recognized that she did not want to be dependent on him for her psychological existence.

In family conversations, she was made aware of the losses and grief her maternal grandparents had experienced in their lives. She understood that her mother too was a good girl who did not burden her parents with her difficulties. Lara felt that hers were small in comparison and that there was no justification or place for her pain. We understood the background to her learning to be there for others and not to demand anything for herself, to provide selfobject needs for others but not to expect that others would do so for her.

The relationship with her boyfriend was going well. Lara felt that it provided an area clear of bingeing and purging. She had been free of symptoms for two months already. She was able to expose herself to her boyfriend and share intimate details of her life with him, and she admitted to having an eating disorder. She was working on herself, managing to soothe and regulate herself, not looking for food as compensation for thwarted selfobject needs. She was at her parents' home on the weekend, felt she ate too much but was unwilling to spoil her clean record. She felt she was in a good place, had found her space and was calmer and more secure in that.

There were difficulties in her relationship mainly because of her boyfriend's difficulty in expressing himself with words. When she told him she loved him, he was not able to declare his love for her and she binged once. She said he gave her acknowledgment but was not prepared to commit to a long-term relationship. She was afraid of losing him. I told her I thought she was afraid of losing what he provided for her, a safe haven, a place where it could be taken for granted that she would be seen, acknowledged and understood. I tried to calm her with my perception that she now had a stronger core that would remain with her even if he left. On the whole, she felt better about her body, terminated the nutritional counseling after 18 months and declared that bingeing was not an option. She was considering moving in with her boyfriend and debated on how to protect her private space in a shared home. She was concerned about being an original artist who thinks out of the box and at the same time being in a long-term relationship without becoming too conservative.

For the first time, she cried in a session. She had been home and had discovered that her father was suffering from depression. Suddenly, she was confronted with the fact that her parents had internal worlds of their own in which all sorts of things took place. She needed her boyfriend to accompany her more on visits to her family, something which was difficult for him.

She had come a long way, expressed fears of becoming dependent on the therapy but also fears of termination of therapy. She requested to come less frequently because of the distance she had to travel to come to the sessions and the pressures of work, and I agreed. She began working with a new choreographer, felt free to bring personal content to the creative process, even content relating to her eating disorder. She was excited, challenged, stimulated, felt herself creative, as an independent source of initiative. In our discussions, she revealed more details of the disorder from her past. The dance enriched the therapy and the therapy enriched the dance.

During the festive season, she went home to her parents and her boyfriend to his. He did not call her during the two-day holiday, and she became extremely anxious. She was overwhelmed with emotion, upset and agitated, unable to contain herself, most unlike her usual self. The discovery of her intense need for her boyfriend was frightening and complicated for her. Lara was able to comprehend the complexity for her of relying on another person to provide selfobject needs, rather than on food. Food was always available while another human being had his own agenda, his own needs, as her boyfriend had demonstrated in this situation. She had been forced to wait, to find a way of soothing herself without his acknowledging presence or voice, his protective shield. Although very difficult for her, her growing ability to do this demonstrated her increasing capacity for self-regulation gained by the process of internalizing the soothing function, through transmuting internalization. Lara's boyfriend had failed her empathically on this occasion, but his usual readiness to be there for her helped her to deal with this instance of his having failed her.

After eight months of no bingeing, she became inquisitive as to how it would feel if she did it again. She was horrified at the ease with which she returned to old patterns of behavior. She told her boyfriend about the binge, no longer hiding it. After this "experiment" she returned to bingeing and purging approximately once a month. Each time, she was able to connect the episode with some emotional cause, to comprehend the thwarted need for empathy and acknowledgment.

She reported a day where nothing went right. She felt bad physically. She went home and cried. She felt disconnected from herself, could not see where the sadness came from. I said that she was connected to herself, could give expression to her feelings, even if they were not clear to her, that she was on the emotional track and did not turn to symptoms to soothe herself. She cried in the presence of her boyfriend, and it felt strange. She saw this negatively. I suggested that something was being set free from the "black hole" buried deep within, the pain which had never found expression. She was able to relate to this description. With her boyfriend, she felt acknowledged. He was able to see her pain, encouraged her to talk about it and would not let her off the hook. She had not experienced this in any other relationship. He was a catalyst for change in her, enabled transformation. She feared losing him. With him, she experienced intimacy in which she did not lose herself and felt recognized.

He became ill while they were travelling together, and she had to take care of him and all the organizational procedures. She discovered she had strengths of which she was not aware. Their intimacy grew even deeper and they began to discuss a shared future. They moved in together. She described their creation of a calm and secure place together. She no longer felt the need to run anywhere, to seek her own autonomous space.

She cried in a session when faced with some financial pressures related to the move but managed to cope without symptoms. I admired her progress. She no longer binged but occasionally purged when she felt full. Life was not perfect, and she realized that maybe she would never be completely satisfied with her body, that there were still issues to work on in the relationship and in her professional development and would probably always be. She felt a pull between accepting herself and striving for more. Her boyfriend was not always sensitive or ready to compromise when she needed that of him. She realized that he was only human and that she could deal with the frustration and not turn to bingeing. She fought with the urge and understood the process better. She understood she was not totally reliant on him and could soothe herself.

With her progress in therapy, Lara became more daring and creative in her work. She began an independent project. She spoke of the need for meaning and depth, for expressing something special, out of the ordinary, something of hers. Her performance was successful, and she was gratified by the experience. I said that there was more room now for her independent center of initiative, more energy for creativity.

She had been in therapy for three years and felt she had achieved what she had set out to do. She knew that she still needed to become more flexible about her diet but felt more balanced and stable in her life in general. Lara now realized the connection between her eating disorder and her emotional life, that it was not simply a habit.

I shared with her my continuous efforts to find the correct words to make her feel understood. She took full responsibility for not being clear. I recognized that familiar place of autonomy. In her view, the work in the therapy was entirely hers. I was the taken for granted selfobject. She admitted that it was important to her that the therapeutic relationship not be too personal or intimate, that it take place in a public institution and not a private one. I recognized that it needed to be in a place that was not mine and did not compete with her autonomous zone.

She was aware of wanting in the past to bring content that she had already processed to the therapy. She had become more open and accepting of the fact that she did not need to know everything by herself. It was very difficult for her when she cried in the sessions. I commented on her preference for intellectual discussion, avoidance of exposing her emotions, her pain, her weakness and shame. I revealed to her that I was moved by her tears, that I saw them as a sign of her emotional growth and maturity.

Because of my vacation, there was a long break until we had our final meeting. She related that she was working hard and that she had had some professional success and felt fulfilled. She sometimes missed bingeing but reminded herself of the ugly side of it. She managed without it. I expressed my admiration for her new coping skills. She said that she was leaving the therapy with more than she had expected to gain. She felt that it was because it was the first time she had chosen herself to come to therapy. She thanked me for my search for the right words and the right timing for the reflections that aided her. She presented me with a book of poetry of which she was fond of and went on her way.

15 The Right to Exist

Laura Canetti

Mary, an Israeli-born woman holding a bachelor's degree in arts, approached therapy at age 27 following a breakup with a boyfriend, which took place approximately two weeks earlier. Mary had suffered from restrictive type anorexia since the age of 16. Until she started her relationship with this boyfriend, she was pretty much balanced; but in eight months of relationship, she lost over 10 kilograms of her weight. Her boyfriend, alarmed by her deteriorating mental and physical condition, argued that he could not deal with her disease and broke up with her. At the time of admission, she also complained about weekly headaches and twitching on the left side of her face. She thought these last symptoms to be connected to stress.

Mary was a chubby girl and decided to go on a diet, since – as she said – she tended to think that unless she was a perfect human being, she had no right to exist. She was amenorrheic, to her delight, between ages 16 and 22. Over the years, her weight fluctuated (in the range of 20 kg). She was bulimic for a while at the age of 19, and once again in her second year of university. A year prior to admitting to our clinic, her weight was 55 kg, with her height being 1.65 m tall. While she was living with her boyfriend, she went on a diet again and reached 43 kg.

Mary was the youngest of three: a brother 12 years older than her and a sister eight years older than her. She describes a pleasant childhood, surrounded by a loving atmosphere and many friends. When she was seven, the summer after she graduated from first grade, she was hit in a car accident. Crossing the road by herself, she was severely hit by a truck. She suffered a severe pelvic injury and was unconscious for two days. Rehabilitation took years, with her family devotedly protecting her and taking care of her. She grew to be dependent on her parents and established a close connection with her brother who treated her like a father. When her brother got married, she was very angry at him and felt like a friend was taken away from her. After the accident, Mary experienced social isolation: although she returned to school quite shortly thereafter, she had no friends, was afraid of the other children and spent most of her time with adults. Studies were extremely difficult for her. She would make an effort and study hard and then hand in an empty examination paper. She says that she was depressed until the age of 18, had suicidal thoughts and was often angry and bitter. Mary blamed the accident for anything that went wrong in her life. She thought that if it wasn't for the accident, she could accomplish much more in her life, referring to her siblings who did very well professionally. She does not blame her parents for letting her cross the road alone or for neglecting the personal injury lawsuit.

Mary associates her anorexia to her desire for perfection and her need of control, which emerged after the accident. During adolescence, she felt different than everyone and was afraid of people. She wanted to prove that she had the right to exist in the world and to feel that she is "worthy," thus she started her diet. At the same period (age 16), she met her first boyfriend, six years older than her. Throughout the years, she was single only for short whiles. After breaking up with her first boyfriend, she had been in a long relationship (age 19 to 26) with a guy to whom she was attracted because of "his aggressiveness." She feels she lost herself within the relationship and that she did not make any decisions because she did not believe in her own power. Mary left him after she realized he did not respect the things she did. Even before leaving him, she started a relationship with a 42-year-old man, divorced with children. She loved him deeply and felt that he was respectful and encouraged her in all areas. In fact, in a closer observation, it turned out that she lived vicariously "through him"; namely, the hangouts he picked became her hangouts, his friends became her friends, his hobbies became her hobbies, and it was only in these areas that he encouraged her growth. Their couplehood was founded upon his choices, and Mary in fact unknowingly deprecated herself in the face of his wishes, feeling that he filled her up. She says that while with the previous boyfriend she was depressed, with the new one everything was more optimistic. She started to relive life through him – only it was his life rather than hers. As stated earlier, he left her after she resumed her anorexic behavior. Mary says that he cannot deal with her problem and that she understands him but is also angry at him for leaving precisely when a problem emerges. Apart from her relationships with men, Mary had no other social relationships. Although she deeply wants friendships, she suffers social isolation to this day.

Mary first started therapy at the age of 19. She was in private treatment for two years, and she feels it helped her considerably regarding the car accident. In her second year in the university, she began another treatment with a psychologist in a public facility. After two years, her therapist moved her to group therapy, in which she participated for two years. She thinks that the group provided her with confidence, especially in her social interactions, but that now it is time to stop and start individual therapy. It should be noted that in both cases, therapy was ended dramatically: In the first case, Mary went abroad and the therapist demanded payment for the time of her absence – Mary resisted and ended therapy. In the case of group therapy, one of the therapists was killed under tragic circumstances and subsequently, the group decided to dissolve.

Mary is a pretty woman, very thin, dressed tidily and sportive-fashioned. She looks much younger than her age. She has no speech disturbances, although her sentences are broken and she switches between topics rapidly. She gives the impression of insecurity and deep anxiety. She speaks openly about her problems, but the moment she starts talking on a particular subject, she tends to compulsively stick to it, and she is extremely annoyed if her interlocutor interrupts with remarks or questions that might derail her from her line of thought.

Mary had been in treatment at our clinic once a week for three years. At the beginning, the core issue was the recent breakup with her boyfriend. She talked about her love for him and her wish that he would come back. She brought up a lot of anger for leaving her when she was weak. She made efforts to improve her anorexic symptoms, so he would have her back. Over time, she realized he wouldn't come back and started to work through the separation from him, with many mood ups-and-downs and many days of depression and longing.

At this point, I tried to explore the problems in the relationship with her boyfriend that drove her to develop anorexic symptoms when she was with him. Despite my efforts to find a connection between the relationship and the disorder, Mary fiercely refused to acknowledge any such link. Furthermore, she emphasized the opposite. According to her, she had the strength to go on a diet precisely because she felt so good with him: "I wanted to be 'hot,' I felt so good I could 'live on air,' eat just vegetables and bread." In this period in therapy, I insisted on discovering the problem in the object-relations level: I thought that perhaps it was the fear of rejection that led her to try and be prettier, or maybe the need to establish boundaries and the fear of losing herself in the relationship brought her to starvation. However, Mary made it quite clear that I was wrong: it wasn't out of distress but out of the strength and confidence provided by this relationship that she started her diet. In her own words:

> [within the relationship] I felt good. For the first time in my life I felt I was living without all this tension of my existence. . . . It was precisely because I felt calm that I wanted to be thin again, thin like I was at 16.

These words made it clear that the core of her difficulties is related to something else, something concerning the "tension of her existence," and that she sought relief through dieting.

This understanding creates a dilemma: Should I be empathetic to her need of the symptom, thereby legitimizing such a pathological behavior, or rather should I ignore the disorder's adaptive aspects in order to present a clear position against the anorexic behavior? I ultimately chose empathy toward Mary's need of the symptom, which allowed her, too, to admit that her anorexia became the only successful arena in her life. Of all the failures she experienced over the years, both socially and intellectually, her success in her diet was the only arena she could feel victorious: "Any kilogram I lost gave me the feeling that 'here, I made it.'" Triumph over her weight gave her a sense of self-confidence.

Two months into therapy, Mary opens the session as follows: "For a while now there has been no progress in therapy because we are wasting our time talking about my boyfriend, instead of resolving stuff." Mary says she is filled with energy and she does not know where to channel it. She has many plans, wants to study many things and knows not where to start. I could think, at this point, that she attempts to deny the pain of separation, that she tries to protect herself, but her will to change the subject seemed to me like a genuine attempt to reach a deeper layer of her relation to herself. She no longer needed me to support her in dealing with the pain of separation. Rather, she needed me to explore other issues, which were more related to constructing her selfhood than building a relationship with someone else. She wanted "to resolve stuff" in order to re-assemble them. In one of the sessions she expressed her intense need to resolve something within herself before she can be available for a new relationship: "I may need this loneliness now. I need to delve deep into loneliness, to get to know it, not because I want to be alone but in order to feel things."

Indeed, Mary didn't "feel things," because something in her sense of self-worth was deeply damaged, to the feeling that her life was meaningless. The meaning of her existence often comes up in the sessions. She says it already in our first session: "I tend to think that unless I am perfect I have no right to exist." Later she adds: "If I live the wrong way, then I have no right to exist." The lack of self-worth is also reflected in death wishes: Mary would have wanted to replace fallen soldiers because they – unlike her – were skillful and could "make it in life." She is concerned with the question of her skills, and she goes down several roads to discover what these skills are, to find a field where she could be "talented."

In the first stage of therapy, she tries to build herself through art. She talks about her feeling that her artistic creation is "stuck" and wants me to help her break this "stuckness." She wants to fulfill herself in the field of art but is uncertain of her talents: time and again she asks herself whether she can be creative or whether she must abandon her aspirations. She speaks of stagnation: she bought the tools to create but cannot approach the materials. She bought a pricey camera but cannot take a picture. At this point, I mirrored her wish to express herself and initiate things that would give her a sense of self-worth. We also discussed the car accident as something that hurt her precisely when she was at a phase of growth and development. Her will to establish her sense of self-worth was also manifested through the creative work: at some point, Mary decided to reach out to a craftsman to learn the trade (which she already studied at university) from scratch. Mary approached him and said: "Listen, I know nothing. I want you to teach me from the beginning. Even though I studied I feel like I know nothing. . . . I purely want to learn the technique, I don't care about design." These statements reflect her inner feeling. The feeling she has no clear self is like the feeling that "she knows nothing." But at the same time, the urge to grow is evident, even if it means starting from scratch. She wants to learn "the technique," that is, she wants to start with the foundations, build her self from nothing. Her desire to build her self is also evident in her endless search for the thing in which she would feel talented and successful. At the beginning, she tries to succeed in art and starts to study with the craftsman. She starts to practice a new sport and gains a sense of strength. A few months later, she embarks on a therapeutic class (alternative medicine), aiming to turn it to her main occupation. After a year, she feels she cannot be good at it and turns to another new field. She quits her job and dedicates herself to learn the new profession with great efforts. But when training is completed and she has to find a job, difficulties emerge and she loses faith in herself. The recurrent pattern is that Mary studies anything with enthusiasm and that studying gives her a good sense of growth; but in the transition from studies to work, she loses her will and feels lost. Her parents, who finance all those endeavors, are desperate and pressure her to do something practical. They intensify my own dilemma: Should I, like her parents, encourage her functional side through interventions that interpret her fear of growth and her desire to stay a child? Or should I let her "play" and legitimize her commitment-free explorations?

The following vignette illustrates the concerns in this therapy: Mary tells me that she decided to quit her artistic endeavors and that she will not meet with the craftsman again.

> I decided to stop the race, to stay only with the things that make me feel good. I suddenly realized that I cannot create there, with him. Although I thought I would want to work every day, I can't. It's been two weeks now that I haven't gone there. I don't enjoy myself anymore.

According to the understanding that she needs freedom and lack of commitment in order to enjoy her craftwork, I said:

> The thing is that you turned something that was previously a pure delight to a necessity, to work. Your will to make this occupation your source of income damaged something. When art ceased to be a hobby for you, you ceased to have fun.

Mary positively reacted to this interpretation, telling me this was exactly how she felt and that she was glad to hear it from me.

At the beginning of therapy, Mary used to speak incessantly, according to a pre-determined plan, without letting me say a word. She wanted me to listen without responding. She never directly resisted my interpretations, but later on, she made a point to explain to me why I was wrong. Of all my interventions, she usually recalled only the questions I asked, which she contemplated at home and used to come with the answer to the following session. In this behavior, she showed me how strong was her need of another person validating her, serving as an accurate mirror of her feelings and only as such. Therefore, whenever I failed to accurately reflect her feelings, she insisted on correcting me in the next sessions. This can be seen as a weakness (thinking over my intervention all week instead of resisting me on the spot), but it can also be seen as a strength. She took an effort to discover her true feelings, and thus succeeded in consolidating her unconfident self.

Mary needed me only as a listener, and that was the case with other people in her life. The need for others as selfobjects was evident: she went to workshops that provided maximum listening from others. When she talks about her boyfriend, it is clear that she doesn't need him as a partner: "I guess I need someone to make it easier for me. I only need the touch of someone, but I don't want to *be* with someone." I mirror: "You need someone to be with you so to encourage you, to appreciate the good things in you." Mary agrees, saying she doesn't want to live with him and "all" she needs is "the touch." She didn't succeed in establishing friendships over this time, among other reasons because she wasn't able to treat others as independent objects. She herself attested to her impatience for others, to her wish to be listened to but inability to listen herself. In her own words: "I like being listened to, but I don't want to hear the reply, I feel like saying 'shut up.'"

At this point, she begins to fear that those surrounding her would refuse to serve as her selfobjects: she often complains that her parents are tired of her, "mom had enough of [hearing me], and both are tired with my intensity." The fear not to be stood by is also apparent in the transference. She is afraid that I will "suddenly betray her." She is afraid that I, like others in her life, will fail to serve as her selfobject because her parents probably failed in this task. It is possible that they didn't serve as adequate selfobjects from the beginning, but it may be the case that after the car accident, when her needs intensified, they couldn't handle the task. Mary's memories validate this hypothesis: she remembers her mother

> giving and giving until she could no longer go on, and she would say to me "I can't take it anymore" and then I'd stop, or I would go on just to spite her. . . . My father couldn't handle the thing altogether.

The failure goes on today as well. Her parents are "tired with her intensity," that is, unable to contain her pain and depression. The boyfriend could not meet the task either and left her precisely when she needed him the most. The previous therapy also ended in failure, when the therapist failed her, requesting payment for the sessions she missed when she was traveling. Finally, the group therapy that was ended abruptly because of the death of one of the therapists also repeated the trauma. It is very likely that these experiences of her adult life were added on top of her early experiences with her parents. This is also the reason why she runs to workshops where she meets strangers: she prefers strangers as selfobjects because the close ones had failed her.

After a year in therapy, progress was evident. Mary started to feel more self-confident, for instance feeling that she talks with her mother like equals rather than having to rely on her. She could also enjoy the compliments she received from others, making progress by the fact she felt people could admire her. For example, in a workshop she attended she related her life story and was complimented for the ways she coped after the car accident. After that meeting, she felt high-spirited. The shift was also apparent in her basic experience of the relationship with me. During the first year, she felt she was a burden to me and that it would be difficult for me to treat her. The turning point took place during one session, where she told me how much therapy meant to her. In the following session, she said: "I told you that therapy meant a lot to me, and I think I saw that you were touched. I think I saw that in your eyes." For the first time, Mary felt she did something good for me, that she managed to make me happy. This experience entails change and reparation: she feels that there is one close relationship in her life where she can be admired, and that she can make someone happy. In another session, I did not respond to something she said and she demanded my response. Such a demand shows that she started to feel safer with me: she no longer wanted just to be heard without hearing the other person – as she still felt with her parents – she was already able to hear another opinion.

In her relationships with others, a change was evident in that Mary increasingly wanted to be at the center, wanted to receive, rather than just serve others. She told me, for instance, that she was working certain days at a store, and another employee who was sick asked her to switch the shifts. Mary wouldn't agree at any rate. Another example: a friend with a learning disability met Mary so she could help her cope. Mary had no patience to hear the friend's story because she wanted to "do things *together* with her"; that is, she refused putting herself at the service of her friend but wanted to enjoy time with her. Mary was delighted with this discovery of her ability to live for herself, and even shifted to the other extremity. This situation gives rise to the therapist's dilemma as to her ability to acknowledge such extreme and often inappropriate behavior. What helped me not to let go of the empathic position toward her need to live only for herself was the understanding that this was a crucial stage for her on her road to building and reinforcing her sense of self.

In the last year of therapy, Mary met a guy who was very patient and knew how to be attentive to her. As opposed to previous relationships, where she completely gave up her self to follow the other, this time she maintained her freedom and her activities and established a much more equal foundation within the relationship. This relationship strengthened her considerably, fulfilled basic needs and reinforced her self-confidence. The relationship also put an end to the loneliness she felt after the previous breakup, and furthermore, appeared to provide her with a fostering environment for her growth.

In the last stage of therapy, most of Mary's concerns focused on the subject of work, and this was the core of the therapeutic work. At the beginning of therapy, Mary worked at a store, until the owner changed and she was forced to quit. She started professional training provided by the Ministry of Labor to acquire a trade that would allow her to make a living. She put a lot of effort in the professional training, and here too there were frequent fluctuations of her self-confidence. We discussed how since the accident she had to put in much more effort than others to accomplish mediocre achievements, and this hurt her immensely. She also talked about her parents urging her, as a teenager, to attend an academic high school, and this might have been an exaggerated demand that caused her great pain. She does not want to repeat this mistake today, so she gives herself a break and seeks to do only what makes her happy. For example, when she went job hunting at the end of the professional training, she entered a competitive market. She could not stand this competition and was distressed, her productivity decreased and eventually she was fired. She was highly concerned about not managing to make a living and being practical. I encouraged her not to cease searching for the right field for her, understanding that she is still in a stage of growth and self-search, and still very far from the stage of doing.

At the end of therapy, the following changes were evident: Mary no longer needed a predetermined plan to talk; she was more communicative and less associative, while making room for me in the conversation and being able to listen to me without feeling threatened; and she managed to put herself more in the center, lived more "for herself" and less for others. She found in her surroundings people to fulfill her needs of support and encouragement and a boyfriend who loves her and cares about her. She is invested in the relationship, but this time while maintaining her activities and her independent life, without the total depreciation of her personality that was evidenced in previous relationships. As far as her anorexia is concerned, immediately after the beginning of therapy, her weight increased to 50 kg, and she was stable at this weight, on the verge of normative, along the entire therapy. Her weight loss was stopped, even though her end weight was still somewhat below the desired weight. The occupational field was still problematic, and she will have to face many challenges until she finds the right place for her. At the same time, she considerably deepened her training in a paramedical profession, and she would possibly be able to fulfill herself more fully in this field. She ended therapy feeling that she gained a lot and that for the time being she wanted to cope on her own. Three months after the end of therapy, she called to tell me she got married.

16 Beauty and the Beast

Eytan Bachar

Anna was 21 years old when she was admitted to our clinic at the urging of her family. A year before her admission, her sister was married. This sister, a year older than Anna, was an object of massive envy and competition. To be "prettier" than the sister at her wedding, Anna imposed on herself a strict diet that practically consisted of an almost total avoidance of eating. The little food she did eat, mainly on Saturday nights, she vomited voluntarily. Anna lost many kilograms, reached a weight 20 percent lower than the expected weight and ceased to menstruate. She was diagnosed with anorexia nervosa, restrictive type.

Anna was the third child in a family of four children. The oldest son was Yonas, then Tessa (the said sister, a year older than Anna), and Danny, who was four years younger than Anna. At the center of Anna's psychic life was the competition with her older sister. The age proximity gave rise to many comparisons between the two sisters by friends and relatives. As far as Anna was concerned, the crucial arena of comparison and competition was their looks. It seems that relatives also stressed the appearance. Anna painfully recalls how she heard her older brother telling a friend that he had one beautiful sister (referring to Tessa) and one "plain" (referring to Anna). Anna herself picked a much more degrading title to describe the comparison of the two sisters: "Beauty and the Beast," the name of the known fairy tale. This reflected Anna's sense that she was as ugly and heavy as a beast.

Anna experienced her mother as a cold woman incapable of giving love and warmth, who did not know how to observe things from her daughter's perspective. The mother preferred the oldest son, worshipping him, perhaps for being a boy, perhaps for being her firstborn, and probably for both. Given his privileged status, his preference of the other sister was well-remembered and particularly painful for Anna. In her experience, the mother preferred the other sister, too. Anna on her part made massive efforts to please her mother: physically – through assisting with housework; socially – through amending small slips her mother had while talking with her neighbors; psychologically – through her constant alertness, always ready to feel if her mother was upset and make up for it. Anna never missed an opportunity to buy her mother presents on her birthdays and on holidays. It was often painful for her to see her mother giving those presents to Tessa, the sister. She experienced her father as more attuned to her than her mother and recalled that he was often available for her when she needed his help. However, these advantages were considered less alluring for two reasons: First, this positive ability of the father was equally implemented in his relationships with all the children, while Anna was hoping for some kind of affirmative action to make up for her mother's alienation. Second, it appeared that the father was reluctant to stand up for one of the children if it could be interpreted as opposing the mother.

The first weeks in therapy were characterized by Anna's hesitation and doubts as to what she called her "dependence" on me. When one of the sessions was cancelled, she opened the following session by saying: "What is happening to me? Am I beginning to feel dependent on you?" When I asked her to reflect on this question, she said:

> It is surprising for me to realize that I have never felt dependent on any person. I was never able to feel dependent on my parents, especially not my mother. This relationship [with me] is my first stable relationship. I think that the first couple of days following our session are in order food-wise, but it is only enough for two or three days. Toward the second half of the week I stop eating, wait for the Shabbat dinner, then throw it up. How would I be able, one day, to transfer this dependence on you to someone else? Whether in a relationship with a boyfriend, or friends in general, it would mean that I have to give up my individuality, the closed door of my room, the consolation and order I gain through preoccupying myself with food. Thus far, what I see in human relationship [meaning the relationship of her parents] is only manipulations, lies and tensions.

I said that I felt that human relations cannot yet compete with what she gained from preoccupying herself with food avoidance. It seemed that she felt relief, but maybe also surprise, by me not arguing with her feelings about food and about shutting herself from relationships.

In one of the following sessions, Anna related a dream in which she stood next to her parents' graves. In her associations of the dream, she said that she felt she could not confront her parents, particularly her mother, and demand what she deserved. She felt that if she demanded presents equally worth of the presents given to her siblings, or insist that her siblings join her in preparations of Shabbat dinner and cleaning afterwards, it might lead to the death of one of her relatives. When I commented that she felt that if she manifests her presence in the world it would seemingly be at the expense of someone else, she replied with a sense of revelation: "It is also connected to my metaphor of the Beauty and the Beast element between me and my sister." When I asked what she meant by that, she explained that she felt it was like a closed system: "If I am the beauty then she is the beast, if she is the beauty I am the beast. Like there is no place for two beauties." Anna repeated this contention several times in the following sessions. In one of them, she added that she sometimes thought that the birth of her younger brother Danny would inevitably lead to the death of one of his older siblings. Regarding the allegory itself, making her the "beast," I offered a comment that later sounded to me with a somewhat cognitive tone: "Even beasts let themselves enjoy food, but you don't." Anna accepted this comment and told me that indeed, to facilitate vomiting, she would imagine "disgusting beasts."

> Now I think about it that my sister and her husband can enjoy so much a dish of hummus with olive oil, whereas I, when the nutritionist suggested to add a sandwich with things that I love so much, thought to myself that I could not indulge myself with such foods.

In this regard, we discussed the notion that by avoiding eating, she does not look for beauty but rather attempts to illustrate for herself that she is unworthy of indulging herself or feeding herself. Over the following sessions, Anna talked a lot about her yearning for the love of her mother. "I feel as if until she gives me back the love that I miss so much, I will not be able to love myself and indulge myself."

After several months of therapy, Anna met her first boyfriend, Evan, who would later become her husband. In one session, she said that Evan, too, does not know how to indulge her and pamper her. When she sensed my surprise (since to me it seemed that Evan pampers her quite a lot), she explained that he did not surprise her with flowers when they celebrated a certain event in a restaurant. My comment that "he did not perform the rituals that you hoped he'd perform" led to the reply: "Call it whatever you want, rituals or not rituals." I sensed she was offended since I did not look at the situation from her perspective and therefore said something that could be interpreted as accepting his viewpoint.

I explained this understanding of mine, and her response surprised me with its clarity and precision. She said in tears:

> This is the only place that is really mine. You are always on my side, even more than I am on my side. I know that Evan has his own needs and issues, but I never thought that in my hour you'd attend to them rather than to me.

I agreed that it was essential for her that I look through her perspective and stated that I understood how painful it was for her when I didn't do it. These clarifications somewhat mitigated the pain and anger, but for several weeks she continued to feel resentment and said that in those weeks her eating patterns deteriorated. As we progressed, it became evident that her reliance on Evan was increasing. We understood that the more she lets go of her pathological eating, the more she turns to Evan and the higher are her expectations that his attention, warmth and love for her would increase. At the same time, it was interesting to see how as her relationship with Evan became closer, the less she turned to superstitions (black cat, broken mirror, etc.) to "soothe and get life together." The bigger Evan's place is in her life, the smaller the place of Tessa, her sister. At this point in therapy, Anna recalled her sister telling her, when she was in the eighth grade, "your clinging to me interferes with my life." Anna's first response to that comment was to think of suicide. "See how quickly I thought back then to give up my place the moment she said it was crowded." She had a dream in which her father told Tessa to take one of Anna's sweaters. Tessa resisted, saying it was Anna's, and the father said, "never mind, Anna doesn't need it and she can always give up." In regard to the dream, she said that she noticed that each time she gains some weight, as therapy progresses, her father joyfully says: "You'll go back to what you used to be – smiley." She said that she didn't like something about this comment from her father. She continued her stream of associations and told me that recently he'd been telling her a lot that she "illuded" others, especially him. For instance, when he wants them to drive together to the countryside in his crossover (his favorite hobby), first she agrees and then regrets it.

> I think that the case is that when he asks me for anything I automatically agree, like any other request of my family. In fact, I hate the crossover, but I always knew how much it meant for him so I said yes. Now, after I automatically say yes, I examine whether I really want to.

The last third of therapy, which lasted for approximately six months, witnessed Anna's fear of losing her brakes. She was afraid that once she starts expressing her wishes, she won't be able to stop: "If I start eating freely I wouldn't stop until I look like a barrel," and "If I met you as frequently as I really want it would be every day." I told her that now, when she starts to want and to express herself, she fears that there is nothing inside her to regulate her behavior – as if she didn't believe that she has developed the ability to regulate her behavior.

> I am particularly afraid how I can transfer my confidence in my relationship with you to my relationship with Evan. If I rely exclusively on him, rather than my preoccupation with eating and not-eating, he won't be able to be there for me all the time.

Gradually, it turned out that there was another aspect to her fears of fully attaching to Evan: sexual attraction and delight of the sexual relation with him, on the one hand, and a sense of stress when they are in bed, on the other hand. In these situations, she did not let him mention her family members, not even a word. She further emphasized that she specifically prohibited him from bringing up her father and brothers when they are in a sexual situation. Working through these fears and prohibitions, Anna's feelings about this area became clearer:

> I was afraid or maybe hoping that since adolescence dad is sexually aroused or attracted by me. I have no real foundation for such a thought, maybe glances that he might or might not give me. I am sure that had I had sufficient love from my mother I wouldn't need to think or look for his attraction to me.

At this stage in therapy, I noticed a somewhat strange behavior upon her entrance to sessions. It was summertime. As soon as she walked into my room, she used to take off her shoes and walk to her place barefoot. When this phenomenon became consistent, I asked Anna about it. At the beginning, she dismissed my question and said that it was simply "summer and it is hot." After a while, my question nonetheless stirred some interest and then she said that in fact she used to walk barefoot quite a lot, and that it had simultaneously two functions: first, it was an attempt to some sort of exhibitionism or a thought of sexually teasing men, especially her father; and the second, a form of asceticism, as she used to do it often when it was cold, or when it was uncomfortable for her. Such "exhibitionism" was allowed since it was not too sexual, so she could practice it also in the presence of her father. Walking around barefoot attested, so she believed (after becoming aware of this in therapy), to asceticism and modesty, traits well appreciated by her father. Anna, of whom such traits of self-deprecation, abstinence and modesty were typical, could easily harness these traits of hers and add them to behaviors she thought would have some sexual "gain," too. It should be noted that once these issues emerged and were discussed in therapy, Anna was quickly released of the sexual tensions with Evan and their relationship was reinforced. Walking barefoot, where it was uncomfortable, stopped. According to Kohut (1977b), the emergence of an Oedipal layer after working through the layers related to harming the self is a very reasonable occurrence. I will jump in time and say that in the follow-ups, a year after the end of therapy, Anna showed up with fancy sandals and told me that as part of what she was capable of giving herself today, she also indulged herself with fancy sandals.

A few months before therapy was finished, Anna married Evan. Since their marriage until the end of therapy, her full remission and improvement were maintained. Her vomiting completely disappeared, and she gradually gained weight until she began to menstruate again. Anna became pregnant and had a baby after we terminated therapy. In the follow-up sessions, she told me that her life, Evan and her baby girl brought her joy. "One smile of Evan, or the girl, is worth a thousand times more than the stupid joy I previously had for any gram I lost."

17 The Right to Need and the Permission to Require

Mira Dana

Maya was 17 1/2 years old when she approached the eating disorders clinic at her own initiative. She was diagnosed with bulimia nervosa, purging type. She has been bulimic for a year, with an obsessive preoccupation with her weight. She is terrified of getting fat and switches between binge eating and voluntary vomiting to periods of fasting. According to Maya, her bulimia started on a five-day "survival fieldtrip" with her youth group. She fasted for four days out of five, and in the fifth she had a full meal, felt sick and threw up. This had started a pattern of fasting, binge eating and voluntary vomiting.

Maya is the youngest in a family of three children. Her labor was difficult, forcing her mother to stay in the hospital for several days for surgery. Maya describes her family as warm and loving, and the relationships at home as pretty good. The parents still love each other after 25 years of marriage. According to Maya's description, this is a healthy, warm and very loving family. Maya's closest relationship is with her brother, who is four years older than her. Her relationship with her older sister is not too close. Her sister is highly introverted and considered to be less of an achiever than the rest of the family.

Maya feels that the expectations from her are high. For example, scoring poorly on an exam will make her depressed for two weeks, even if no one explicitly tells her it is unsatisfactory. She fears letting her parents down, and consequently she fears disappointing everyone around her, as well as anyone who knows her.

Socially speaking, Maya is popular and has many friends, but in fact none of them are really close to her or know much about her. Some of her friends may think they know her, but usually she doesn't like telling other people about her true feelings, her problems or her pains, not even to the closest ones. Eating, food and preoccupation with body shape and weight fill her time, and they bear the entire burden of feelings and problems. This obsessive preoccupation conceals the problems and the painful feelings with which it's hard for her to cope.

Maya's father is a clever and rational person but emotionally closed off. He tends to lose his temper easily and represses many things, he doesn't express his emotions, his communication is indirect and he is anything but a homely person. He likes the outdoors – nature, sports and traveling, goes out a lot with his friends, doesn't like to be at home and spends minimal time there. Maya's mother is stubborn, emotional and strict about her values. Maya's parents do not spend time together – they are busy with their distinct activities, but they do so out of their belief in freedom and love. Maya has an anorexic-bulimic relative in her family. Her family does not have shared meals – each of the family members eat whenever it suits them.

In an overall observation of the treatment, it's hard to say that Maya was persistent attending the sessions. She was often late or completely failed to show up, sometimes without notice.

For the first session, she showed up wearing a blue shirt with children's prints on the front, her long haired pulled back. She was ten minutes late for the session. At the beginning, I presented the therapeutic contract: duration of the sessions, duration of the treatment and the fact that the therapeutic hour is hers and she can talk about anything and use it as she likes. Maya then started to talk about a new boyfriend she met. The relationship progressed slowly, and she was anxious about the dependence she felt toward him. She felt that when they are together, she occasionally manages to eat normally, but in his absence, she eats and vomits. When she does eat with him, she feels fat and pushes him away. At such times, she does not want him to touch her at all, particularly not her belly. The relationship is founded on her fear of dependence and dread of him leaving her if she shows her desire and affection for him. The boyfriend, on his part, acts like she bothers him and like she's a nuisance to him. Her response to that is to act indifferently toward him and then he comes back to his senses and begins to desire her.

I did not say much at that session, apart from a few words about how her dependence frightens her so much, like it was some kind of entity she must hide from herself and from the world, and that by pushing her boyfriend away from her, she realizes what she fears the most. She rejected this interpretation and in fact behaved most of the session like she was talking to herself, or like she doesn't really mind who it was she was talking to or who else was present in the room with her. She must have been very afraid, unknowingly, of her dependence on therapy, of her relationship with me, and thus she pushed me away, or whoever I was supposed to become – namely, a very important figure in her life for the year to come.

Indeed, our relationship, as she later called it, was characterized by going back and forth; that is, she was frequently late or failed to show up at all – "ditches" as she used to call it – demonstrating her fear of dependence, of closeness, of true relationship with me where she might be seen as she really is; in other words, as she truly and internally sees herself.

Maya started the next session with a long description of her school and her female classmates. She had been screening them all with a comparative eye, with the exclusive criterion of being fat versus being slim. She always examines herself based on her appearance, always in terms of fat or thin. I told her that it seemed that she always looked at herself and her appearance through the eyes of the people surrounding her – through the eyes of the boys in her class, saying that she is the fairest of them all, or comparing her looks to the women she sees around her. I told her that she needed constant reassurance from the outside and that she did not look at herself and her condition from within.

She talked about her anxieties as to the direction she'd take in her studies: Would she succeed? Would she get good grades? She detailed a long list of anxieties regarding her functioning in school, for instance, her wish to be popular. I said it was natural to have anxieties before school begins concerning her schedule, classes, teachers and friends. But it seemed, I said, that along with these anxieties, she also expressed her anxieties about her treatment, since her therapy began when school began, and her fears in this regard were similar to those in regard of school – what kind of relationship we'd have; whether she'd get "high scores" in therapy; would she succeed; would I consider her popular; what direction would therapy take; and how much she'd need to open up in therapy. Maybe, I said, there was another fear, connected to the one discussed earlier in the session, that through understanding and insight, she'd end up eating "normally" and lose her opportunity to use her body for comparison and compliments. Maya used the rest of the session to describe her anxieties about the therapy, both because of my interpretation and because of previous psychological treatments she experienced that led nowhere, as she put it.

For many sessions afterwards, Maya was going back and forth between closeness and distance, between attempts to talk about herself, her pain, her feelings and the fears that make her move away from me. For instance, in one session, she talked for the entire session about suicidal thoughts she had throughout the week. While the way she talked about it did not scare me much as to the actual realization of these thoughts, I nonetheless understood it was an attempt to show me that she has a painful, desperate and hopeless part inside of her.

Maya did not show up for the following session, and I interpreted it as her saying that this closeness, exposure and dependence are too difficult for her and are frightening her. I later found out that after that session, she ate and vomited much more than usual. It is common that the patient tries to convey something through her eating, to communicate feelings she is unaware of or has trouble to express.

Along the entire treatment, Maya speaks highly about the therapy. She describes how much she feels connected to me, how she became dependent on therapy and how much she loves the challenges it puts her through. At the same time, she has a constant need to please me. Those compliments may very well be another way to do that, even though she is clearly being honest.

Throughout therapy, Maya's ambivalence about her right to receive and her right to enjoy herself is apparent. She does not believe at all in her right to receive and her right to fulfill her needs. It is also apparent that she does not believe in her right to receive anything from me or from therapy; therefore, she misses appointments, showing up for one appointment but missing the other. The core problem expressed through these absences is the question "How much am I worthy of treatment? How much can I trust a human selfobject, Mira?" On the one hand, Maya showed her wish to come to sessions, complimented therapy and made it clear that it was important to her. On the other hand, she could not believe she was worthy of another human being (rather than substance) who could fulfill her selfobject needs. She did not believe she could actually trust me to always be there for her (as long as therapy goes on).

Maya knew well the confidence she drew from trusting food, which is always there, never fails her, never abandons her and seemingly fulfills her needs, relieves her loneliness and soothes her pains. She found it hard to invest this trust in someone else, a human being, although it is possible that such person would be there for her. It was difficult for her to feel worthy of such fulfillments of needs, and this was one of the struggles she had to face in therapy. This struggle was most evident in the apparent play between presence in sessions and absence from them.

After several months in therapy, Maya began to feel better about herself. She began to work for a living alongside her studies, and she felt better about who she was and what she was doing. At the same time, and probably not coincidentally, anger toward her mother began to rise to the surface. For example, she was angry that right when she feels better and more connected to herself, her mother starts to interfere with her life and limit her choices. It was as if the moment she attempts to find a positive identity for herself, some independence and autonomy, she feels her mother is pressuring her to retreat from this positive place.

At the same time, her boyfriend sent her a love letter from overseas, and she panicked. She felt it was like a bank note she would have to pay when the time comes. She didn't know what she would do if he would still be into her when he comes back from his travels because that would mean she would have to be in the presence of a human being who treats her so nicely – a person who is close and accessible.

Maya's father began to play some new and more important role in her life, which threatened her mother who found in Maya the answer for her loneliness. Maya's father began to fulfill Maya's needs better and to a larger extent; like taking her out to a festival when she wants it, rather than when he pleases. He tried to understand what she needs and to meet those needs, at least partially.

However, things were more complicated in her relationship with her mother. Maya became attached to her and found it difficult to separate toward independence. Maya's mother on her part also found it hard to let Maya become independent because of her loneliness and her distance from her spouse, Maya's father. When Maya's father witnessed the close mother-daughter relationship, he became detached and distanced.

These dynamics between Maya and her parents and between her parents themselves were brought up in one of the sessions, in which she told me she was smoking, and that was a secret between her mother and her, of which the father did not know. She said it was something that connected her and her mother. When I asked whether there are other secrets of which the father is not aware, she gave the example of being no longer a virgin. This bond with her mother excludes her father and perhaps substitutes for something in the relationship between her parents. It is as if the relationship between Maya and her mother is somewhat founded on the exclusion of her father, of him being left out, and like something in the parents' relationship is reduced because of such secrecy and exclusion.

The small amount of food Maya eats (still 300–500 calories a day) demonstrates her inability to enjoy food, and in a broader sense, her overall inability to enjoy herself. She feels that she's not allowed to enjoy herself, and most of all, that she's not allowed to enjoy food. Any delight always raises guilt feelings and pangs of conscience. For example, whenever she goes out, she must stand for several hours in front of the mirror and excruciate herself and those around her with questions about her looks from the front, rear and sides. These hours are stressful for everyone.

She is by no means allowed to fulfill her needs. Not fulfilling her needs is also existent in her relationships with men and therefore in sexual relationships. In this regard, too, she feels that sex is forbidden; thus, she must never want or need anything while having sex.

In another session, Maya started with a story on a school fieldtrip that took place a week earlier and the huge amounts of food she ate during it – food she had not allowed herself to eat for many years. Maya argued that 70 percent of the girls in her class eat and vomit. She also described a very common situation for women and girls with eating disorders: before the meal, she can perceive herself as thin, and afterwards, even if she ate only minor amounts of food, she inevitably sees herself as fat.

Later Maya told me about a fight with her closest friend and said that although she felt secure with this friend, and although nothing particularly concerning happened in this fight, she feared that her friend would want to end their friendship. To interpret this event, I used my own relationship with Maya. I associated the event with Maya's sense of abandonment and despair regarding the end of the therapeutic relationship. We have already come a long way together, and the end is in sight – it can already be sensed. Maya remained with the question with what color would the forthcoming termination endow the sessions that are still left and the relationship that still existed.

Maya did not show up for the next session. In the following session, I compared her absences to her eating pattern: she shows up for one session and misses the next – like eating and immediately throwing up.

Like other relationships Maya finds and chooses, our relationship entails something scary for her and she finds indirect ways to deal or avoid dealing with her fears. In her relationships with men, her indirect coping mechanism is to date two men simultaneously or find someone who is leaving the country soon, a married man or inaccessible in any other way. In her relationship with me, her indirect way of coping is through her absences, being late for sessions and her long monologues during which she does not relate to anyone present, like talking to the mirror.

Maya's eating pattern began to change in that period and within a month has radically transformed. She finds herself eating endlessly without vomiting. This is quite a common phenomenon for those who stop fasting or vomiting, let themselves eat anything and "discover" the foods that were thus far forbidden and now became permitted.

On a practical level, I tried to understand what Maya meant when she said "eating endlessly" – quite unsuccessfully. But on the emotional, psychological level, I nonetheless symbolically translated the change of pattern by comparing it to an image of Maya sitting in a cafeteria with one cucumber on her plate, looking at those around her with envy, on the one hand, and with superiority and contempt on the other. I did not forget the feeling she then had. The feeling that she needs nothing or doesn't deserve anything – neither food nor people. Everyone around her keeps on running, connecting to each other, talking, communicating and loving, and she watches them from the outside, with the one cucumber on her plate, symbolizing her miniscule needs. In light of this memory, the change of eating pattern signals a shift in her relationship to herself, to her needs, because her current way of eating entails recognition that she needs something. She does not know what it is that she needs, she is unaware of the nature or essence of this need, but she at least lets herself feel that she needs *something*. Therefore, she turns to food and lets herself eat without vomiting.

As already mentioned, Maya allows herself to recognize her needs through eating – she lets herself eat, even "forbidden" foods, and feels that she wants and needs to eat, a feeling she previously avoided through vomiting and fasting. This fact is in itself a symbolic expression of the beginning of Maya's recognition of her needs.

We discussed again our relationship that would eventually terminate and the intense fear it raises for Maya and that this was the reason for her back and forth – showing up and then missing sessions – instead of maintaining a steady relationship with me. This way, it was more familiar and less scary.

Later we talked about the way she must somehow ruin anything she enjoys, like work, therapy and relationships. Anything joyful is at the same time scary, so she must destroy anything that is good and pleasing, just like she does to food through vomiting.

Maya's family lives in a small three-bedroom apartment with one bedroom for the parents, one bedroom for Maya's brother, and the third for Maya and her sister, several years older than Maya. In this arrangement, Maya clearly has no privacy. In fact, she has no corner of her own. For a long time, she has been asking to close off the balcony so she could have some kind of a room for herself because no doubt she is too old to share a room with her sister. Her parents agree in principle but postpone the issue in practice. At this point in therapy, the fights with her parents got more frequent, both about the room issue and about other issues. The more Maya found herself, the more she began to demand, to need and to stand up for herself, the tougher the domestic situation became.

Maya's request for privacy, her wish for a room of her own and the capability and courage to fiercely insist on them are significant milestones in her personal and therapeutic development. Following one of the quarrels about the room issue, which once again ended in vain, Maya started a "hunger strike," as she called it. She began to fast, protesting against having no room of her own and claimed that she would go on fasting until a room with some privacy would be arranged for her.

At this session, Maya was very sad and desperate. In some kind of a philosophic speech, she presented her feeling that whatever she does or will do is pointless and useless. This included high school diploma, academic degree, work, entertainment and finding a boyfriend, which in her eyes, "all was the same, all for nothing."

At that point, I tried to draw her attention to the timing of this hunger strike. I reminded her that two weeks ago, we had a meaningful conversation in which we talked about her needs. I reminded her of what we said, that maybe now, when she lets herself eat much more than that single cucumber, she is also making a symbolic statement about the fact that she has needs that she could no longer deny. I told her that she must have reached the recognition that she was not beyond the human need for relationships, care and food. And here, precisely at this significant timing, right after making such a statement and after taking in and enthusiastically accepting this interpretation, she immediately enters the same place of fasting; and through fasting, both practically and symbolically, she once again denies any sign of having needs. I suggested that perhaps the previous session's statement and insight about the very existence of her needs, about her very right to be a human being, suddenly scared her and she retreated to her un-needing existence; that is – she dared to articulate her need for a room of her own, and when she was rejected, her protest once again took the form of self-deprecation, this time through a hunger strike.

It was clear beyond doubt, to me and Maya alike, that a room of her own was an essential and vital need at her age. It was also clear to both of us that the actual and practical inconvenience of the present situation was unbearable. But at the same time, we also knew that it was only a symbol, only the cover story; that even if an actual room was arranged for her, the underlying conflicts would emerge onto the surface in some other way. That is, it would be in a similar statement taking a new form. It was therefore important for her to understand what she was saying through her hunger strike in order to bring the true conflict up to the surface. This is her conflict concerning her needs, and it was the core of the room fight and the consequent fasting. Maya was terrified of disclosing her needs, of the explicit discussion of her being a human being and of the fact that she has needs, and this terror drove her to protest and deprecate herself through fasting.

In the following session, Maya described at length her concern about her heavy weight and her lack of elegance and told me how painful it was for her. She mentioned the fact that she was just weighed and that despite limiting her food intake to one salad at noon for the last three weeks, she still hadn't lost any weight. She weighs 60kg and it is frustrating when she sees her friends eat anything and still manage to stay lean and lightweight.

It was obvious that this conversation about her weight, while charged, was a substitute for the real talk, to avoid touching the real pain, which was so difficult to talk about so it was brought up only ten minutes before the end of the session. Indeed, a few minutes before the end of the session, Maya started to describe a fight she had with her father two weeks earlier. The fight started when she wanted to leave the house after having an argument with him. Her father said, "you are not leaving anywhere" and physically prevented her from leaving the house. The argument proceeded until it eventually culminated in a painful and humiliating situation in which her father sat on her and beat her hard while shouting and threatening her. Her older brother, her closest and most beloved person in the world, heard the shouting and entered the room. He did not try to stop her father; rather on the contrary, while her father held Maya down and continued to hit her, her brother held her legs to allow her father to beat her more freely. Her mother also entered the room at some point, told her brother to stay out of it and left the room at once. Her father spilled out in front of her brother, her mother and Maya herself all of his complaints about her egocentricity and her egoism, while going on beating her all along.

Obviously, we had no time to discuss this incident beyond that. I said it had to be significant that she told it just at the end of the session and that it was probably also the reason why she did not show up last meeting and also considered quitting therapy. Maya responded that it might very well be connected, although she did want to talk with me about the fight when it happened. We agreed that we had to get back to it and that we'd have more time in the following session.

Predictably, Maya did not show up for the next session. A week later, she talked in detail about pneumonia that prevented her from coming to our session. She also talked about her relationship with her closest friend, who was the only person with whom Maya could feel truly wanted, loved, safe and pleasant. She talked about feeling very fat, vulgar and ungraceful. We said that in the mirror Maya was seeing her inner figure, depending not on her actual weight but on her feeling toward herself and that her friend was like a special mirror that reflected her good parts, and that only there, with that friend, she lets herself look upon herself as a positive person. I suggested that what she sees in the mirror are her needs, those parts toward which she feels disgust and contempt; in the mirror, they take the form of fat and ugliness.

We discussed her needs, her emerging understanding of how she prevents herself from relating to them and how only now she is beginning to acknowledge their existence and essence. In most sessions now, she talks about her body weight – how fat she feels. She feels that aside from me, all other people in the clinic try to "brainwash" her with the message that if her weight is okay, then she is okay.

The next session was deep and meaningful, and we discussed her needs at length and in depth, perhaps with a new insight: how she really ignores her needs, how she really fails to recognize that they exist and how much she is considerate of others' needs. We also talked about her eating pattern, which is the symbol of her lack of attentiveness to her own needs. We then proceeded directly to discussing her role in her family and the relationship between her parents. Despite their mutual complaints and protest, her parents still live together. For example, her mother goes on saying how much she would rather be with someone romantic and emotional, but in fact she keeps staying for many years with a rational, practical and unromantic man, while complaining about these very traits.

The entire talk evolved around Maya's role in the relationship between her parents. At first, she served as a selfobject for her parents; company to her father but mainly to her mother, a woman who sought a close, attentive and comforting human figure. Since she could not find such figure in her husband, she turned to Maya, saving herself the disappointment and inevitable confrontations with her husband. Maya relieved the mother's loneliness and spared her – with her closeness and attempts to please – the pain of deficiency and absence. Perhaps Maya's most significant role was to separate the parents during fights and mutual anger and to serve as a mediator and conciliator. Slowly, Maya began to reflect on her needs, to put herself at the center of her world and retreat, a little each time, from the role previously undertaken. When Maya began to invest in herself, the mother was left alone to face the father, which caused increasing conflicts.

The less Maya "protected" them from anger and fights, it seemed that the dam broke loose, and the parents began to bitterly confront each other. A noteworthy point that only in retrospect became quite apparent is that in her initial intake interview, when asked about her parents and their relationship, Maya described an idyllic picture of a warm and loving family. She described a very close relationship between parents who still love each other after 25 years of marriage, respect each other and seldom fight.

There were probably two reasons for this description. The first was Maya's need to see things favorably and conceal the problems underneath a nice and pleasant façade. The second was that things were in fact calmer and less problematic because of the significant role Maya undertook in the family dynamic. When Maya realized this and slowly began to free herself of this role – a very dramatic, however gradual, shift occurred in her home environment and in her parents' relationship. The fights became more and more frequent and their distance grew more apparent and explicit. Until about a year after Maya's therapy ended, they went through a serious crisis that led to total separation and ultimately to divorce.

In the following session, Maya talked at length about her relationship with her parents – her father who lately was constantly angry and yelling at her while trying to control her life, and her mother who was "tormenting" her. Maya recites the session in which we discussed her family role as a crucial, intense and significant session for her. She felt she understood something highly important about her relationship with her parents and with herself.

In the last third of the treatment, I felt stuck. In the supervision group, I realized that I was overemphasizing transference interpretations, interpreting as an external, experience-distant object. That is, I stressed too much the relationship between Maya and myself: almost any material she brought up was worked through both on the level of the event itself and on the level of our relationship as separate objects. Later I shifted the emphasis away from our relationship and attempted to connect to her from her own perspective. In the sessions, it was manifested through my attempt not to interrupt, as much as possible, with her sometimes endless flow of speech. I connected to the actual experiences that she brought and her perception of me as near to her experience allowed her to connect to the feeling that preoccupied her. For example, when she talked about the emptiness she felt after letting go of the bulimic symptoms, the peer group suggested not to interpret it from without, in terms of the therapy's progress, but to connect to her difficulty facing the loss of a previously gratifying preoccupation.

One of the most apparent outcomes of this change was that for several sessions, Maya talked about what she had been through, her feelings, her thoughts, etc. At that point, an entire session could go with only Maya talking from beginning to end, and I am only listening, saying nothing until the concluding line of "okay, we must stop now." At this period, Maya is extremely bothered by fat and food. In the sessions, she defines herself as fat and as "a cow," saying that she hates her body. She sits on the couch in my room with shorts, saying that she feels like she is actually spilling out over it. She feels much internal confusion in this period. Each session witnesses another story. At one, she talked about caring less about her body, and in the next, about her feelings that she is fat and ugly. So many external and internal changes had occurred in her life, and she still holds to her body like it was fat, to avoid fully acknowledging those changes.

And then, a few sessions before the end of therapy, something happened that made me understand a certain aspect of the relationship between Maya and her mother. In the session, Maya talked about caring less about her body. She no longer looks for bones as an indication of fat, she feels less obsessive about food and cares less about not being able to fast, she eats much more and she does not excruciate herself as she used to about food and about her fat. The energy she used to devote to her obsession faded away and now she basically feels exhaustion and emptiness. "Life does not happen to me," she says. Nothing happens to her but rather life goes by her. She tries to show me how lacking and empty her life is. She no longer vomits, although she still eats very little and counts the calories of many foods she takes in.

The surprising part was that I felt "stuck" in the therapy. In my peer group, I talked about feeling helpless, paralyzed, like we did nothing in therapy, because it is ending and Maya still feels emptiness, exhaustion and that life goes by her. The group asked me why I can't be proud with the changes and improvements that took place, why I don't give credit to the symptomatic changes and the changes Maya underwent and why I feel so "stuck." I was told that Maya showed a clear symptomatic improvement, which was accompanied by intrapsychic change because Maya is so happy trusting her own judgments. The group members also added that it was clear that once you get rid of a heavy symptom, you feel empty, lacking, exhausted and in pain and that Maya felt that because previously it was the symptom that constantly preoccupied her. When she "breaks up" with the obsession and has nothing else to preoccupy her all day long, she finds herself empty, exhausted and lacking.

What I realized in the peer group was that at this point in therapy, I did to Maya exactly what her mother did to her throughout her entire life. She never acknowledged her pain, she wasn't empathic and she, too, was detached of Maya's flow of speech. Maya had to cry out her pain for someone to recognize and hear it. Bulimia was her scream. A child needs her parents' empathy like oxygen. Maya, following her experience with her parents, in fact does not believe that anyone can truly listen to her. She is so terrified by the chance that her listener would not be empathic and fail to understand her, so to prevent the pain and the trauma involved in the lack of attentiveness, she talks frenetically, immobilizes the listener and paralyzes her. It was my own empathic failure that I could repair, and so I did. The reparation was to acknowledge Maya's emptiness, fatigue, which was so authentic, without feeling paralyzed and helpless.

And then we reached the final session. In this session, Maya talked optimistically and very warmly. She summarized therapy and all its aspects in a very personal and positive manner. In the following, I bring the spirit of this session and then accurately quote Maya's response on the treatment conclusion, which she wrote four years later, as I was writing this chapter.

Eating-wise – Maya reports she started to eat. She even eats in the presence of others, which had she never dared to do before. She goes out to a restaurant with a friend – regular meal with no dietetic food. Eating there evokes guilty feelings and she feels bloated afterwards, but then it goes away and she is left with the food in her stomach and with the feeling, and she simply goes on. She also eats "forbidden" foods, that is, eating improved considerably and it is fair to say it became normal.

Her feeling toward her body was the aspect least changed in therapy, the most difficult aspect that gave her the hardest troubles. She knows she is not fat, yet she nonetheless feels that way.

In all other aspects, she now feels she has needs, knows she is allowed to satisfy them and that she is allowed (a little, not much) to be with someone who loves her and treats her well. Indeed, she knows that her relationship with guys is an issue she feels she hadn't quite handled.

She says she feels that she is afraid of our separation, but in any event, she feels she no longer needs the dependence on me and on my positive feedbacks because she thinks she accurately analyzes the situation and knows she is okay. She feels that she knows where she stands and that her self-analyses and self-understanding are much more objective and true now. She independently recognizes when her self-analysis is right, and the source of her concerns or discomfort; she knows how she can reach a practical solution and also recognizes the instances she tends to "feel sorry" for herself. She feels she can give to herself, that her weight is stable and that her eating is normal.

Despite her dissatisfaction with her looks, Maya ceased to vomit, fast and use laxatives, and she is doing well in her high school final exams. She said: "They say that for every 20 minutes of talking there are 7 minutes of silence. I don't recall even one minute of silence in all the hours I was here. So maybe we'll have one hour of silence." She feels she does not wonder too much, that her helplessness is gone and that she can manage her own business.

Maya feels that her improvement during therapy was gradual rather than abrupt, and in fact she even feels a little bit strange that she dared to say that with so much confidence because she always used to think she is "unworthy" and deserve nothing, and suddenly, she feels she does deserve, that her achievements are important and that she can appreciate them. She has a greater sense of self-worth and recognizes that she's allowed to have good things in her life.

In regard to her relationship with her parents, she says that in fact the fights weren't that harsh, other than a few exceptions. The relationship wasn't exceptionally good, either. She feels that she doesn't think that much about her relationship with her parents because it doesn't preoccupy her as much. She lives her own life – doesn't want to be bothered and doesn't want to bother them. Maybe in the past, she was concerned about the overattention they'd given her. She says that as far as they are concerned, she is okay, although they still fail to accept her feeling about her looks. In fact, she says, everything worked. Therapy worked beyond the practical achievement that brought her to eating normally and to letting go of her food obsession. She is annoyed with her current sense of emptiness, frustrated for having to pay the price of giving away her preoccupation with food. She says that the way she thinks is still distorted in relation to her appearance, but in all other spheres, she is capable of standing for herself and needs no external validation. She needs no mental dependence anymore, not on me and not on conversations that would validate her positive thinking of herself.

She points out another aspect for which she feels she pays no price and she likes that. She feels independent in her thinking, that she is okay and entitled, and for this she pays nothing in terms of depression, and it's even nice for her. She says that it's like things are divided into two, the symbolic side and the conceptual side: the conceptual side includes the things that are good for her; and the symbolic side – what's good for us, her caretakers, namely, the ceasing of vomiting and the normal eating.

The symbolic side is okay for her as well. That is, she is very glad for not having to deal with food obsessively, but she says it is a little cruel to take away the content she gained from this preoccupation and to add a few unnecessary pounds because it made her feel bad. She fears her army enlisting and the "final price." She really hopes this would be the final price she would have to pay in terms of gaining weight, since she already feels bad about it and doesn't want to go on gaining weight.

She asks: "How did you have the patience never to yell at me, never to get angry at me? You have never said to me 'this makes me angry' about anything."

She says she loved our conversations. She loved to talk with me. The fact that I never told her I was angry at her made her feel guilty, but it also had a positive impact. She says:

> Way to go for bearing me, bearing the parts I was pissed off and didn't show up or gave you a notice. Your restraint and the calm way you make your comments to me is something new. I don't know how often I'll meet something like this in my life, but I know for sure I hadn't experienced it before. I don't want to sound sentimental, but you'll always have a special place in my heart, and the period of our meetings is extremely meaningful.

As I stated earlier, I hereby quote Maya's description of therapy as she wrote it four years after it terminated, when I wrote this chapter:

> I hated the clinic. I hated going there every week and being weighed. I used to weigh myself with my back towards the scale so not to discover that I gained another 100 grams. I hated fighting with the nutritionist whenever she tried to set up a meal plan for me. I hated the cold empty rooms in which I used to see Mira. I knew I was different than the daily landscape there. I was never underweight. Even when I stopped eating, the lowest weight my body reached never put me in physical "risk." And then it stopped. I stopped losing weight. When I first started therapy, I had already gained 3 kg from the lowest point and I felt the fattest in the ward. I was anorexic. And bulimic. And slim. This I know today. I approached the clinic at my own initiative; when I felt helpless after several months that I used to vomit all day long whatever I dared eating. I panicked. I stopped eating. I used to drink water all day long and have an apple or a low-fat yogurt at night. Simultaneously, I started putting more effort in my studies – hours over hours, obsessively. I lost weight rapidly. 8 kg. I felt stronger and better. At that time, I met a man 21 years older than me and fell in love with him. His mature figure and age gap only attracted me more to our sick relationship. He was about to get married – not with me . . . and all I wanted was him to be the first man I would have sex with. Nothing else. And so it was. And everything seemed magical and fairy-like since a fantasy just got real. Even the loneliness and depression that followed couldn't undo the feeling that I made a fantasy coming true and that it was "awesome." After that, I made it a habit to hang out only with people older than me. I was looking for considerable attention. I loved "controlling the situation." To this day I love controlling the

situation. When I was sixteen or so I started to calculate calories. I had a friend who was the expert on calories and I looked up to her. And she was thin. Way too much. She was anorexic and swept me in to this "trend." This is another thing I know today, in hindsight. The youth group, that was the center of my world, ceased to excite me. The new school I moved to had taken its place. I gradually became detached from my old friends in favor of my new classmates. I began to work in a small bar and met a group of people over 10 years older than me. This thrilled me and made me curious, but I felt I had to change in order to be liked.

My best friend was anorexic at this point, and I couldn't recognize that. I only knew I envied her. She seemed to me slim and fragile, more beautiful than ever, and I wanted to compete with her over attention. During the school year I stopped communicating with my classmates. Only my best friend – who went to school with me – stayed close and I kept the latent competition who is thinner. When I could no longer fast, I started to eat huge amounts of food. Every day. And throw up everything. Every day. And use laxatives. Every day. The decision to approach the clinic was also made following my friend, who started therapy there herself. I remember the dread I felt on the first day. They wanted to put me in group therapy. I felt I would lose the center, where I love to be. That I would disappear among the other stories and cease to be special. That I would have to share attention with other people. And then it was decided to give me individual therapy after all. I don't remember the first session with Mira. I think I told her how everything started and what I was going through up to that point. I loved talking about myself and Mira was attentive and seldom talked back. There were times I didn't show up. I didn't want to be weighed and I didn't want to disclose myself to anyone. I felt that if I would continue therapy as I was supposed to, all my problems would go away and I would stop being so disturbed and special. The entire home circled around me. My parents lost their peace of mind. My older brother, my dear brother, hated me with all his heart. He thought that I was just being spoiled. My older sister didn't try to understand in depth. In the talks with Mira I disclosed how I lost my virginity, that I was attracted to older men. The games I liked to play – always date several men simultaneously so everything would seem complicated, and ultimately push them all away and stay with myself. Mira speculated that I do not give myself a chance to be loved. That in accordance with rejecting all my basic needs – food, the company of my peers, pleasure, etc., I also deprive myself of the right to be loved by someone who can really invest in me. I only enter hopeless relationships, as if I know I wouldn't get what I deserve so I wouldn't commit "a crime" – and let myself feel good. I used to take each talk with Mira home and reflect intensely about it. Each time I got a new perspective into my mind and tried to analyze it anew. I hated myself so much that whenever I let myself feel good, I would evoke a huge need to punish myself for it. Therefore, I scarred my body with ugly burns, I distanced myself from my parents' warmth whenever they tried to show understanding and patience, I looked for ways to destroy anything good that I could have and please anyone else around me but myself. In eleventh grade I used to work at a pizzeria. I would study and work, and eliminate any possibility for free time. I kept measuring the limits of my strength. Then I met a young man who was a friend of someone I worked with. We went out together a few times, talked about all kinds of topics and I understood he was looking for my company. I immediately shut myself to him. Each time I pushed him away diplomatically. After two weeks he went on a long trip abroad. I felt a huge relief. Each time I got a letter from him I would feel uneasy and hate the moment we met. Because he really wanted me. And I knew it and it freaked me out. Because it is "forbidden." I used to complain to Mira that he doesn't let me go even when he's overseas. That he keeps showing his interest and that I don't want him. The day Mira brought up the issue of "family dynamics" changed everything. Not at once. It was a gradual process. Mira suggested that my parents, who did not get along well, do not expect much of one another, and when they do – they tend to get disappointed. My older sister also never lives up to the expectations and it's like she is past the stage she needs to prove herself. My older brother was in the army and he's the only son so he was always treated more tolerantly. And I, the youngest, was left to live up to all expectations that left all other family members unsatisfied. The more I look at my role in the family dynamic I realize that my role is the biggest since I conclude I have to "fill in all the holes" – perfectly excel at anything; school, appearance, work, and at the same time – never ask for anything so to not be a burden. This, in general, was the idea. And it made me realize that things were very much like this suggestion.

I did not leave the clinic healthy. No miracle happened to me and I didn't regain my wisdom and started to eat healthy and balanced meals and think that I am a charming creature who deserves much happiness. I was still confused and unhappy, but I had the tools to cope with at least some of the feelings. I left mainly because I had to join the army soon. To this day I don't think that everything is resolved, or that I am completely "normal." There is always some thing in my head that never goes away but keeps on bothering me. I can't point to it exactly, I just know that nothing turns my world upside down and makes me obsessive anymore. And that I find the world a calmer place, offering me many things that I should and I am allowed to taste. Literally. I would never ever forget the last day. When I sat down, the hour with Mira seemed too short. And I talked with more optimism, like I already discovered the solutions to my problems. I know I lied to myself a little, but I definitely knew I had the strength to go out and fight. Before I left, in the very last minutes, I stated with a smile that I was going out with my man, who returned from abroad and never lost his hope, and kept on courting me until I agreed to receive anything he could give me. And I felt happy. I hugged Mira and felt somewhat awkward know-ing that it was over. That I am on my own. . . . That she wouldn't listen to my heart anymore. That she wouldn't get a little upset any-time I don't show up for a session. That she didn't know we were together for eight months. That I love myself. Deeply.

18 "When Someone Believes in Me, I Can Start to Believe in Myself"

Inbar Sharav-Ifargen

In this chapter, I describe my encounter with a patient suffering from anorexia (restrictive type), whose "fear to occupy space" amounted to starvation on the verge of death. Forced hospitalization was required to bring her to therapy and to actively create room for the very possibility of her physical and mental existence.

Michelle, 19 years old, was the oldest of six children in an Orthodox Jewish family. She was involuntarily hospitalized by a court order for her life-threatening weight (BMI = 9.5). The court determined in its decision that unless she is hospitalized, her parents would be declared as guardians and force her into admission. Prior to her present condition, Michelle suffered from an eating disorder of infancy; difficulty weaning from breastfeeding was followed by days of fasting, and over the years, by restrictive and selective eating with no delight of food. Michelle demonstrated rigid behavior in other domains as well, including difficulty in free play and social interactions. Her fierce resistance to changes or diversity in food led the family to avoid challenging her in order to steer clear of confrontations.

As a child, Michelle was repeatedly hospitalized in pediatric wards for her severe anorexia, all involuntarily. Any weight gain was possible only through using the feeding nasogastric tube. Since long and excruciating hospital admissions brought no progress, she was defined as chronically ill. Her doctors reached an agreement with her that she would be discharged whenever she reaches a target weight, which was much lower than the acceptable norm but was not immediately life threatening. Michelle said they understood that there was no chance to achieve change and agreed with her that she could give up on menstruating and reaching her full potential height. At the same time, however, she was highly motivated to maintain her scholastic performance. Michelle is bright and reached high academic achievements during and in between her hospital admissions.

When she reached the age of 18, Michelle discharged herself and tried to maintain a steady job, while gradually losing weight. Her parents, who supported her all these years and were positively involved in her treatments, were exhausted by years of forced hospitalizations and fearfully observed her dangerous deterioration. They painfully felt that there might be no other choice but to walk her to her death. However, when they felt the risk of death becoming concrete, they found the strengths to approach the court applying to be appointed as her guardians. While her parents could describe her as charming and energetic, they arrived at the ward exhausted, feeling like post-traumatic veterans with scarce hope for improvement. They felt that Michelle was sucking all of their energies out like a black hole and that she ruins the family life. They were terrified by the possibility that she'd move in with them again. Michelle's mother said that she felt Michelle was living "through her," explaining that she couldn't bear it because her own parents also did it to her. She was married at the age of 18 and immediately went through prolonged and excruciating fertility treatments, as she felt was expected from her by her religious community. Michelle was born after a difficult pregnancy, in a complicated and exhausting labor. Her parents described her as a difficult child, persistent and stubborn even before she was born, and the narrative of the painful impregnation and labor was told as an evidence of Michelle's strong-willed character. They described that her strong presence and stubborn facial features were apparent already in her ultrasound photos. She was born with high sensory sensitivity and was difficult to comfort as a baby. They felt they needed to attend accurately and uncompromisingly to whatever she needed, and this was the only way that everything could be alright.

The developmental background suggests that Michelle's mother did not have a good experience of a primary selfobject, making internal room for her existence, but an intrusive selfobject who persistently attempted to live through her, and who had to be rejected for her to survive. This experience had probably contributed to her own difficulty to provide her daughter with a space inside her. The way she experienced Michelle even before she was born, as insisting on making it difficult for her, and as strong, opinionated and stubborn, undermined her ability to hold the full potential of Michelle's existence, first inside her, and later in the world.

Michelle started her hospital admission being fed by the tube, extremely angry about the deprivation of her freedom and hoping to quickly reach the minimum low weight she was used to and be discharged. The ward's staff, too, thought her condition to be chronic, with no chance of achieving any change for a patient whose entire identity evolved around her anorexia and resistance to therapy, with rigidity and elements that seemed to persist from infancy. Michelle's parents feared early discharge but were also afraid, in light of past experiences and her legally adult age, that it would be inevitable.

Except for her refusal to eat, Michelle was vital, and after some physical recovery she took part in all the ward's activities, maintained her personal care and beauty routine and expressed her wish to return to work. At the beginning, she expressed no interest in psychotherapy, saying that all past therapies were forced and unsuccessful and that she wants to live her life alongside her eating disorder. When we started therapy, Michelle manifested no curiosity about her condition and was repetitively preoccupied with the technicalities of her difficulties at the ward and her preparations to apply to court in order to discharge herself. When I suggested that she might nonetheless want to use the therapy to make some changes, she resisted. She said that the entire team of doctors who knew her well understood that that was it and no change could be made. She insisted that she had to be discharged soon and that it was too bad that we didn't know her and didn't respect the past contracts agreed upon. Michelle's talk at this stage was technical, generic and repetitive, generating a feeling that it's impossible to truly get to know her or relate to her. However, along with her strict adherence to her symptoms, Michelle had gradually begun talking about her frustration of her life. While she aspires total control over anything, including her body, she finds herself helpless facing constant disruptions because of the forced hospitalizations, and totally dependent on her family and medical staff. She was hurt by not being seen as a human being because everyone focused only on her weight. Gradually, she could begin to recognize that along with her wish to be known, there is a great fear of getting help, leaning or trusting anyone human, beside herself and her symptoms and that in fact she was trying to avoid a deeper relationship.

At this point in therapy, it was very clear that she was relying on her food avoidance and the rigid preservation of control over her body to provide her selfobject needs, in a manner that gave her a sense of worth and pride, as well as something consistent and forever reliable, contrary to a human selfobject who may fail her. I could sense that there was a part of her desiring change but that the fear of change paralyzed her. She felt this was the only way she knew herself, and that gave her confidence. It was apparent that she was afraid of being more in touch with powerful and unfamiliar emotions emerging from within and that each time a greater emotion was emerging, she would retreat and resort to her repetitive talk about the hospitalization and discharge conditions.

Alongside my feeling that it is difficult to make a meaningful contact with Michelle, which was boring and frustrating at the beginning,
something about her also enchanted me: a tiny girl determined to fight
the whole world. I thought how it must be painful and frightening for
her to be a little girl with no adult around her who is able to confront
her and share her fears. I wondered how it was possible that everybody
seemingly gave up on the possibility that she would develop, reach
puberty, menstruate and lead a full life. Against all odds and contrary to
the sentiments of both the family and the other staff members, a strong
feeling emerged within me that this is unbearable, that we must not
give up, that there is a chance which I must fight for and that I, deep
inside, can envision Michelle coping with her immense fears and continuing to grow. I therefore conveyed the message that I understand
how terrified she is by her prospects of change and growth but that
I think she shouldn't be given up on; that the contract that suited age
13 does not necessarily suit her now, when she is more mature, and that
I believe things must be revisited; that I feel that we must not give up
on the chance that she reaches puberty, develops, starts menstruating
and embarks upon a mature, rich and independent life in which she
would actualize her dreams to study and grow. Her reaction suggested
that even though she was careful to show her resistance and anger, she
was also surprised and even touched by my position, and that my words
found an echo in her heart. She said she didn't think it was possible, that
it was also too terrifying and unfamiliar but that she appreciated the fact
that I thought so and maybe there was something to it.

It was then that our therapeutic relationship began to deepen. It seems
that the restarting of selfobject needs in the transference began when
I made space inside myself for Michelle's potential coming to being,
and seeing her as someone who can exist in the world, take up space,
courageously cope, search for her way and continue her growth. This
provided Michelle, over time, with confidence to start listening to more
complex voices inside her. Alongside her feeling that she is the only
one to know what's right for her, she felt humiliated by her dependence on everyone, and a wish emerged to be able to direct her life more
sophisticatedly.

At this stage, while still in low weight, Michelle began to try and
face her fear of diversity and change and to dare experience new situations, like eating foods she hadn't eaten in years. When she succeeded,
she felt proud, powerful and in better control. In therapy, she began
to acknowledge that she has been frozen for years within her eating
disorder and began to express her will, along with the fear, to break
free. My effort to align with her goals and wishes and to suggest that

there is a way to make it happen, perhaps in a-not-so-scary way, was experienced by her as an attempt to connect to her point of view, rather than dismissing anything that was precious to her and that she holds on to. *Mirror transference* was salient at this stage. Michelle felt seen in a way she had never been seen before and found that she can see in her therapist's eyes a look that is pleased with her, recognizes her strengths and admires her progress and insights in a way that enables her to develop her ambitions, to feel that there are things inside her that she would like and could more fully realize.

When we started to explore together the way she grew up and her relationship with her parents, Michelle said she remembered nothing from her childhood and immediately retreated with suspicion. She experienced this exploration as blaming her parents, said she wasn't looking for anyone to blame, that her parents indeed made some mistakes but that was human and that they were always trying to do good. I said that it was obvious that her parents loved her and were always making positive efforts but that her words suggested that in her opinion, there was always someone single to blame and that it was always her. I added that in her perception, she was the one who was always too difficult, stubborn, impossible, and I thought that wasn't fair to see her like that, that it was important to observe the broader context of her growth and development. This phrasing seemed to reach her. She felt that her perspective is respected rather than fought against but that she is still fought for. She started to openly express her frustration of the adults in her life constantly giving up on her, and in a particularly touching moment, she said: "When someone starts to believe in me, I can also start to believe in myself." Slowly, the thought began to emerge that maybe, after all, she can reach normal weight and proceed to a rehabilitation halfway-out program. It seems that the initial reactivation of the need to grow that began with my own ability to make room inside myself for her potential to exist, revived the potential core of existence inside her.

It was hard for Michelle to let go of her severe anorexia and emaciation, and she didn't want to feel that she was giving up on her anorexia only because of her fear of leaving the supportive ward she got used to. Feelings of contempt toward herself emerged, fearing that she might be weak, letting go of her principles and letting others affect her in a manner that doesn't suit her. In therapy, I encouraged her to continue and examine boldly what does and doesn't suit her. I mirrored her growing strengths. In the past she felt so penetrable, felt like anything could come in and influence her, deprecate and delete who she is, thus she had to block everything by a firm armor. Today, when she is getting stronger, a certain space starts growing inside her. She can begin to take things from outside and check herself, what does and doesn't suit her, what can be left inside and become a part of her and what can be evicted back out, all out of her own choice. Simultaneously, she dares to experiment more diverse eating and richer social situations. Going home for the weekends, Michelle exercises independent eating, and alongside accepting her need of a supportive rehabilitation framework, a strong wish to return home emerges. Together, we could contemplate her wish that after years of hospital admissions, she would be able to go back and be a child coming home and completing the course of her development. Her parents, who received counseling during her hospitalization, were less anxious and also enjoyed Michelle's progress. They felt that they, too, with the therapeutic counseling, can begin and form hopes and faith that Michelle can develop and recover, what they never felt before. They were happy about her home visits over the weekends. However, they were also terrified about the possibility that she would return home permanently with no rehabilitation program and that things would go back to square one, and they again would have to experience familiar helplessness facing the possibility they might have to watch her dying. Michelle talked in therapy about her paralyzing fear. In certain situations when she tried to take some first steps in various experiences outside the ward, she felt that although her parents supported her, in fact they were more terrified than her, in a way that didn't enable her to relax. It seems that during that stage, Michelle experienced her therapist as more calmly confident in her abilities, as being able to see that although she now faces new and scary experiences, whether practical or emotional, she is now able to cope and to be less avoidant, to succeed and even grow stronger, notwithstanding the fear.

Idealizing transference is apparent at this stage of therapy, reflecting the need to be in the presence of a figure who is experienced as big and supportive, and merge with this figure in a way that endows confidence and comfort. This gradually enabled a developmental process, in which Michelle felt more confident, peaceful and pleased with herself and her ability to cope with what was previously deemed as unbearably dangerous. Michelle used the therapy to work through her pain about her parents' inability to contain the anxiety of having her home, despite the improved relationship and her strong wish to go back home. Slowly, she began to acknowledge and accept her need of a residential rehabilitation program. Her home visits on the weekends, along with the understanding that actually moving back home is inappropriate, allowed for a new experience of a more mature and multifaceted relationship with her parents, which could be enjoyed by both parties. Gradually, Michelle had reached normal weight for the first time in her life, and it enabled her to apply to a residential rehabilitation program. Her discharge was not free of concerns, but she was determined to continue her process and cope with her fears. Her fear of listening to her inner world, to recognize and connect with more powerful experiences and emotions was still tremendous. For example, Michelle preferred to adhere to a strictly fixed meal plan, rather than listen and recognize sensations of hunger. The prospects of sexual development were considerably frightening, but even such thoughts were beginning to emerge, along with the ability to refer more fully to emotional complexity in the family, including feelings of frustration, anger or envy. Nevertheless, a more open relationship with the family continued to establish, making way for a more complex emotional communication. Michelle was discharged and moved to a rehabilitation program, where she managed to continue her progress, to pursue employment and academic studies, while maintaining normal weight and eating habits.

Some concluding thoughts: Michelle, a patient with an eating disorder and many difficulties since infancy, experienced long hospital admissions since childhood, with the risk of dying from anorexia. What can be the foundation for such a severe pathology? The etiology of eating disorders brings together many aspects, including family, environmental and psychological factors. I suggested that in Michelle's case of severe anorexia, there is a possibility of a primary injury, in prenatal and early life stages – a deficiency in the selfobject's ability to make internal space for the patient's coming-into-being, which undermines her potential and practical ability to take up space and exist in the world.

Kohut, referring to early life development, referred to the stage preceding the formation of the nuclear self, as a stage in which the child exists only as a potential concept in the mother's mind. "A developmental process which may be said to have its virtual beginnings with the formation of specific hopes, dreams and expectations concerning the future child in the minds of the parents, especially the mother" (Kohut & Wolf, 1978). This does not mean specific content expectations but that the mother constitutes the baby, namely, holds the full potential of embodiment for the baby's coming-into-being self. This process begins in early life in the encounter of this potential being with the actual baby, and the holding of the baby's continuous existence as an actual self in the eyes and the minds of the parents, even in that early phase in which the baby herself has no experience of existence and continuity.

Kulka (2005) broadened Kohut's conceptualization and developed the concept of "virtual self" and its importance as the primary foundation for the development of the nuclear self. Kogan (2011) also writes that in the beginning of life, the parent provides what she terms "selfobject of virtuality" for the baby, thus holds for the baby the association between being and not-being. According to Kogan, it is impossible to be born without a space to exist within a significant other. This function continues along life as part of the empathic matrix, in a way that holds a sense of continuity, the sense that someone essentially knows you, beyond that specific action or another. A human being without such space within another human, feels discontinuity, lack of hope, withdrawn from the course of time. It seems that the notion of selfobject function of virtuality may shed light on the therapeutic process with Michelle, and the way in which she could feel she was beginning to believe in herself and her existence, when she felt, in therapy, that there was someone to believe in her and essentially hold her potential existence even before she did. Kogan titles this kind of primary transference occurring in this stage *"virtuality selfobject transference,"* stressing the special nuance occurring in this primary phase that is related to the very beginning of existing in the mind of a selfobject. She further states that although such a transference occurs to a certain extent with every patient, it would be extremely dramatic in patients who are more archaically wounded.

I found that in cases of severe anorexia, like Michelle's, it is often possible to detect and identify the resonance of an early failure in the way the patients were held in their mothers' mind even before birth. Typically, it is a situation in which the mother was not emotionally available to hold her daughter's potential existence in her mind. There can be ample reasons, like an unwanted pregnancy in an unsupportive environment, or a particular stress such as death of a significant other. I mean, of course, cases of significant pathology in the parent's self, not any immaturity or normal ambivalence held in a "good enough" manner. In the case of Michelle's mother, it is reasonable to assume that her own developmental failures prevented her from experiencing herself as a center of independent experience and emotional existence in the world. Thus, she was unable to provide such a foundation for her coming-to-being child, Michelle.

Understanding the essential injury in these areas may also constitute a basis for conceptualization of the therapeutic process and transference dynamics in some cases of severe anorexia. A crucial factor for the reactivation of selfobject needs in the transference is the ability of a selfobject to internally create a space for the patient's coming-to-being self to exist. This is how it happens before life begins and this is how it should happen in the self's renewed attempts to recover. When Michelle's consistent sense of existing inside me has been gradually established in the transference, she was able to reconnect with the origins of life, and from that point on, she could see her future disclosing.

I will end with Michelle's words upon the end of treatment, in which I was touched to find such a vivid echo of the progress of the potential of her existence within me:

> I thought this hospitalization would be just like all the others and stay at a technical level. But to my surprise I find myself for the first time in my life at a normal weight and on my way to a rehab program. Who would believe it?! The answer is "you." You didn't give up on me even when I already gave up on myself, maybe you truly saw something in me that others had missed, or failed to recognize through the thick black curtain the disorder generated in my life.

19 "I Don't Want to Make It to 20"

Analu Verbin

I first met Eleanor ten years ago, as a fragile 19-year-old girl, when she was admitted into the psychiatric ward at Hadassah University Medical Center in Jerusalem. She was diagnosed with anorexia nervosa at the time; however, her eating disorder took on many shapes over the long time in therapy. I have had the privilege of treating Eleanor for ten years since that admission, through her time in a halfway-out facility for patients with eating disorders, and later on in my private clinic in varying frequencies, depending on needs. Today Eleanor is 29, married and a mother of a one-year-old son, halfway through graduate school. I still see her once a month or two for maintenance.

It is almost impossible to conclude ten years of therapy, while still allowing the reader to feel its essence. Rather than giving a full and comprehensive case report, I will touch the central developments through some illustrative vignettes, highlighting certain aspects of self psychologically oriented therapy. In particular, I would like to point out the development of her selfobject needs over the years of therapy along with the transformation from archaic to mature forms of selfobject transference.

Second among five children in a religious Jewish family, with four male brothers, Eleanor's personality was a mixture of aggressiveness and passivity. Indeed, she explicitly referred to a duality when she described her high school years: at home, she was quiet, docile, helpful and caring; in school and in her youth group, she was hot-tempered, rebellious and confrontational.

Eleanor's teenage years were marked by two traumatic events. The first was her father's death, due to a heart condition, when she was 13. Described by Eleanor as a violent, aggressive and often abusive man, she never missed him. However, from that point on, Eleanor took an increasing part in maintaining the household, helping her mother, taking care of her younger brothers, cooking and doing other house chores. She would later tell me that it was at this point when she realized that her "role in life is to help mom survive." The second event was her mother being involved in a severe car accident, followed by a yearlong rehabilitation process. Along with severe anxieties and fears brought by this event, Eleanor undertook the lion's share of taking care of her mother and the house. She didn't attend school at all that year.

Most of her childhood and adolescence, Eleanor was overweight, but it was only around 17 when it started bothering her. She then sought nutritional counseling for the first time. At 18, she left home for national service and was assigned to a prestigious but highly demanding position, located far away from her home. A first major depression episode occurred, accompanied by a severe weight loss. Because of her mental condition, she was reassigned and later discharged from service. Her depression prevailed, along with the weight loss – all in all Eleanor lost 30 kg over one year. When she returned home after her discharge from service, she began to binge and vomit frequently.

Eleanor was admitted to the psychiatric ward when she was 19. Despite her severe eating disorder symptoms, the staff was more alerted by her severe depression and suicidal thoughts, several times amounting to concrete plans. "I don't want to make it to 20," she said in her admission interview, a phrase understood at the time as expressing her fear of growing up and separating from her mother.

The first few weeks of therapy were frustrating for both of us. Eleanor was anxious and severely depressed, wandering about in the ward like a terrified, lost child. She seemed afraid of anyone, and in the weekly doctors' rounds she used to stand feebly in the corner, as if turning to the wall for support, and could barely utter a word. She failed to meet the demands of her meal plan, and her weight continued to drop. In therapy, it seemed that interpretations did not reach out to her and she could hardly fill the time of the session.

Several weeks after Eleanor's admission, a coincidental technical error had left us with no consulting room for our session. I suggested to conduct the session in the balcony adjacent to the ward. As rain started to fall, we were forced to sit next to each other on the balcony's stairs. I then noticed how being physically close to me allowed Eleanor to relax, like a baby soothed and comforted by her mother's close presence.

This incident allowed me to recognize Eleanor's need of merging with me (Kohut, 2011) for emotional regulation and soothing and shed new light on her difficulties to bear separation and distance. It seemed that even language itself – interpretations and verbal conceptualization – entailed distance (Winnicott, 1965b). This understanding, together with my evaluation of Eleanor's limited strengths and the significant concern of self-harm, led me to favor validating and consolidating her self. Stressing experience-near interpretations over confronting her with her aggressiveness from an experience-distant position (Kohut, 1979), I was consistent with this approach even at the face of risky behaviors on Eleanor's part, which concerned and irritated the staff and me.

Special emphasis was given to experience-near conceptualization of her suicidal thoughts and anorexic symptoms. For example, when Eleanor told me that she'd rather die than be a burden on her mother, I said, "at some points you feel it is better to completely disappear, just not to add an extra burden." Slowly but steadily, Eleanor's increasing confidence in the therapy became apparent and brought about the emergence of curiosity and introspection. Eleanor could speak more openly about her fear of growing up, of leaving home and leading an independent life. Most of all, she was terrified of losing the close connection with her mother, if she "dared" to leave home or withdraw from her family roles. As I reflected and acknowledged these fears, her suicidal thoughts disappeared, together with her vomiting.

However, when Eleanor began to spend short weekends at home, after she made progress and symptoms were reduced, she was having trouble balancing between caring for herself and the family's demand to help her mother and brothers. When she went home for a longer holiday break, she could not stop vomiting, and upon her return to the ward, she restricted her food intake and once again lost weight.

Shortly thereafter, I completed my term at the ward and moved to the outpatient clinic. Nevertheless, thanks to the ward's and the ED team's willingness and flexibility, I continued to see Eleanor. The "system's" willingness to bend the rules in order to meet her needs was experienced by Eleanor as a surprising and meaningful gesture, and our therapeutic alliance was reinforced. She attributed this decision to my power and status in the ward and she called me "a magician." While I felt tempted to break this illusion, I also understood this as idealizing transference (Kohut, 1971; Sands, 1989) and acknowledged its therapeutic value for Eleanor. Her feeling that she was being taken care of by a powerful figure who acknowledged her needs, and furthermore, was willing to use those powers to meet her needs and to provide her with continuity of care, was new and transformative.

Indeed, this marked a new phase in Eleanor's treatment. She was determined to take advantage of her time at the ward and to move on. There was no trace of the scenes that were so frequent in her first months at the ward; and even the experienced nursing staff commented astonishingly that "this is not the same Eleanor." I believe that she then began to internalize some of the strengths and psychological structures she had attributed to me up to that point (Kohut, 1968). She no longer needed to merge with me, and less archaic forms of selfobject transference could develop. Most significantly, she was determined to face the challenges presented by the meal plan and gradually managed to regulate her anxiety and discomfort around eating. It appeared that she could use my empathic echoing of her difficulties, along with my recognition of her determination and strong will, to control her urge to avoid eating or to vomit.

In our sessions, we stressed her difficulties to eat, and especially the difficulty to share her feelings, to "ventilate" or to cry at the dinner table. This opened the road to discuss the death of her father for the first time. Eleanor recalled how she felt during the *shiva* (Jewish mourning week), where she was not allowed to cry. I said, "there was no room there for your own pains or fears because you felt you had to take responsibility and not make it harder for your mother." By gaining room and legitimacy to talk about these feelings, Eleanor was filled with memories, which became more and more complicated and traumatic as we dived into her family dynamics. A richer, however complicated, picture of Eleanor's family was now available to us in therapy, and in turn enabled us to better conceptualize and validate Eleanor's experiences. Eleanor's capacity to contain conflicting feelings was growing, and she was able to express anger and frustration along with love and attachment.

For the first time, Eleanor was able to contemplate leaving home for the sake of her recovery, and she accepted the staff's recommendation to move to a halfway-out facility. For the first time, she also talked, quite embarrassed, about her academic and professional aspirations, in a social science field that was unusual in her social milieu and was not accepted or supported by her family. Perhaps similar to me, she wished to gain academic education and become a professional woman. I welcomed the seeds of Eleanor's growing self and encouraged the motivation and interests that began to emerge.

Eleanor was discharged from the ward after eight months, when she reached her target weight, and subsequently moved to a halfway-out facility. She was fighting hard to continue our therapy, even though it now meant long rides halfway across the country and paying for it herself, since I then left the hospital for my private practice. Eleanor eventually succeeded to convince the new staff to let her continue therapy with me and took much pride in this success. I welcomed her warmly in the new setting and mirrored her achievement and her newly acquired power to fight for her needs.

However, fight seemed to be a key word during her first months in the new halfway-out facility, until Eleanor was able to truly believe the facility staff's sincere concern for her. In self psychology terms, she could not believe that other people were willing, once again, to step up and fulfill selfobject needs for her. She kept asking: "How is it possible that you make all these efforts for me? How is it possible that you care so much?" Gradually, Eleanor adjusted to the new facility's demands, although she still found it difficult to approach staff members for help. She was well-liked by the staff, even though from time to time she had some confrontations with them, which reminded us of her rebellious side that also called for recognition and legitimacy. It was crucial for Eleanor to realize that she could be consistently and sincerely cared for even when she is not totally obedient. I witnessed, and reflected, how this stable and consistent environment provided by the facility allowed her to get in touch with her inner world, along with the ongoing effort to maintain her weight and normal eating. In therapy, we touched painful memories of her childhood home environment that was filled with chaos and terror, and together we searched for the right words to accurately relate to her experience.

Stability, however, was undermined by these painful contents and by the external demand to fully function at work and in her studies. Eleanor prepared for her SATs, but the more she progressed toward completing this task, the more weight she lost. She restricted her caloric intake and once again resorted to vomiting as a means to regulate anxiety. It seemed that any progress in the real world was intertwined with regression in her ED symptoms. I offered Eleanor this interpretation, suggesting that her symptomatic regressions were her response to growing up and occupying more space in the real world, but my interpretation seemed to arrive prematurely and was felt to be experience-distant. Eleanor kept losing weight, which led to further despair and depression. I resonated with her experiences of desperation, frustration and failure, while making great efforts not to let those experiences flood me as well so I could continue and mirror her achievements and progress, too. At the same time, I was concerned about questions of time and pace, what was the right pace for Eleanor. I understood her wish to study and work as a positive manifestation of a developing self, but I was also afraid of change that was too rapid that would lead to collapse.

Eleanor, too, was preoccupied with questions of time. A recurrent theme was her frustration with the time she "wasted" compared to her peers, and she tried to stop the flying time. After particularly stressful days, she avoided going to bed, "to prevent tomorrow from coming, and losing another day." Echoing this experience, I reflected "you want to grow at your own pace, the pace dictated by the world outside is too fast." I also extended our concrete time frame, thus embodying my understanding and acceptance of her need for sufficient time. Acknowledging my efforts to find the right time frame and right pace for her, Eleanor gradually legitimized and accepted her "different" pace and refined her ability to recognize it and to more accurately respond to it.

Excitement and vitality began to reemerge as Eleanor started her academic studies and found a job as a counselor for youth at risk. She earned warm feedbacks and felt enthusiastic about her activity. However, when time came to leave the halfway-out facility and take another step toward a fully independent life, Eleanor was once again petrified and quickly resorted to her eating disorder symptoms, until finally dropping out of university. Two years into therapy, again we were facing depression and despair.

At the same time, as we began our third year of therapy, another significant event occurred: I got pregnant. Within the variety of emotions I experienced, there was also fear of leaving Eleanor at this particularly stressful period. Maternal leave may be seen as a major empathic failure but against the backdrop of an otherwise empathic relationship, it is also an unmatched opportunity for a significant therapeutic progress.

I therefore chose to disclose my pregnancy to Eleanor quite early on, certainly earlier than to any other patient, so to let us work it through and prepare as much as possible for the interruption of therapy. Indeed, in the following months, we were immersed in the contents raised by my pregnancy; and no less intensively, planning and reflecting on my maternity leave and the ways to preserve the therapeutic relationship during this period. While I planned to resume work immediately after the mandatory leave is over, Eleanor was afraid that I would disappear and fail to return to therapy. Furthermore, given her family tragedies, I guessed that Eleanor deeply and only half-consciously feared my sudden actual death. Her anxieties increased and threatened to take over. I wanted to promise I would not abandon her but was also afraid to do so, as obviously I had no guarantee that everything would be okay.

Kohut's concept of emphatic failure became highly useful for me at that point. It allowed me to view my maternity leave in a more positive way and acknowledge its potential of transmuting internalization for Eleanor. It thus helped me to manage our working through of my maternity leave. First and foremost, I mirrored the inevitable absence and Eleanor's sense of empathic failure. We both knew that no matter how I cut short my leave or offer alternative communication methods, there would still be some time during which I would be unavailable for her. It was perceived as even harder given her planned leave of the halfway-out facility.

However, my willingness to admit the failure, and my empathy for Eleanor's concerns and angers, brought out great relief. Eleanor found it reassuring that I acknowledged and legitimized her complicated feelings, and she was able to begin and discuss her fears of death and abandonment. I asked Eleanor how she would like to keep in touch during my leave, and for several consequent sessions, we formulated together some configuration of email communication to be maintained during my leave. The more time and effort we dedicated to this almost-concrete issue, the more Eleanor was convinced that I took her needs seriously. Accordingly, she could empathically and responsibly attend to these needs of hers, without devaluating them on the one hand, and without developing a hysteric, anxious or depressive response, on the other hand. She also began to believe in her ability to actively influence her own life.

My progressing pregnancy was raising a wide array of conflicting emotions for Eleanor, often confusing and sometimes embarrassing for her. She was switching between curiosity, excitement, anxiety, envy, anger and guilt. I legitimized all emotions, empathically reflecting them from an experience-near stance. At the same time, talking about her "here and now" emotions allowed a lively and open talk about similar emotions she had known from the past. Specifically, Eleanor's worry about my health and her need to protect me made room for a thorough and effective exploration of her functioning as a selfobject.

Simultaneously, outside the therapy, Eleanor was planning her upcoming year. She successfully applied for another academic program and won enthusiastic feedbacks in her job as a youth counselor. I acknowledged her achievements and mirrored her growing capacity to choose how to shape her life and to effectively act toward her goals. She still had difficulties eating but she maintained a normal weight and constantly improved her ability to communicate her difficulties and reach out for help.

When I returned from my maternity leave, Eleanor had undergone some significant changes, posing new challenges for her. She moved out of the halfway-out facility into a shared apartment, where she was expected to start and to lead an independent life. She began a new academic program, entailing many public speeches and presentations, which raised many concerns. Notwithstanding the fears and hesitations, she was gradually able to take up central roles in the program and work through the emotions that accompanied this growth. After discussing at length her conflict between "being nice" to people and promoting her own interests, she concluded: "This is probably my present challenge – to find the balance and know that I can be nice to other people and help them, without stepping on myself in the process." She finally let herself live fully, and while she was still preoccupied by food and weight issues, she was able to regulate these feelings without compromising her normal functioning.

In the therapeutic relationship, I discovered that Eleanor could bear the experience of separation from me, which was also apparent through manifestations of anger and frustration. She was able to confront me and express her irritation when she felt I didn't understand her, and she no longer treated me as an ideal "magician" who could read her mind. In fact, I felt that this early form of idealization transformed into her ability to recognize the same qualities in herself. She was proud telling me that she provided advice and consultation to her friends and enjoyed her own wisdom and strength. Furthermore, not only could she now bear experience-distant interpretations, she explicitly asked for them, saying, for example, "suppose you didn't know me, what would you think?"; and she had repeatedly shown me that she could bear such interpretations and continue to work on them by herself. Finally, she began to look critically at her tendency to serve as a selfobject and eventually could envision letting go of this seemingly eternal position.

Whereas Eleanor's eating disorder symptoms had for the most part disappeared after three years of therapy, we had continued to meet on a weekly basis for the following three years. During these years, I was privileged to see Eleanor through completion of her undergraduate studies, through falling in love, moving in with her boyfriend and eventually marrying him. While all these meaningful events make for intriguing vignettes, it is beyond the scope of this chapter to describe them at length. However, it is significant that through these challenging events, she only very rarely resorted to vomiting as a self-regulation mechanism; and even then, these were typically single occasions whose emotional triggers were easily discerned by her.

After Eleanor's wedding, we both felt that frequency of sessions may be decreased to reflect her growing independence and her growing reliance on her spouse to fulfill her selfobject needs. I continued to see Eleanor twice a month for an additional two years; and in the last couple of years, we meet once in a month or two, usually when she faces a particularly stressful period or a new challenge. I see her ability to reach out to me when she feels she needs it as a testimony both to a well-established trust in a human selfobject, and to her ability to be attuned and attentive to her emotional needs. Throughout this period, Eleanor gave birth to her firstborn son, while maintaining a steady professional job and graduate studies.

During the treatment process, the idealizing selfobject need has transformed from an archaic need to literally merge with an idealized selfobject, in the very early phase of the treatment; through the need to associate and identify with it, "this is *my* ideal, magician, therapist"; to a long and sustainable relationship of empathic echoing that has taken the place of the initial merger. Similarly, the mirroring selfobject function has transformed from zero tolerance for any distance, thereby bearing only experience-near interpretations, to the ability to tolerate and then welcome experience-distant interpretations; and eventually the capacity to interpret, understand and regulate emotions and behaviors by herself.

The last time I saw Eleanor, while I was already in the process of writing this chapter, she said upon leaving what I find to be a remarkable manifestation of transmuting internalization: "In the past I had to write down what you were saying to me in order to make good use of it. Now it is enough for me to think about it and know the right way."

References

American Psychiatric Association. (1980). *Diagnostic and statistical manual of mental disorders* (3rd ed.). Washington, DC: APA.

American Psychiatric Association. (1994). *Diagnostic and statistical manual of mental disorders* (4th ed., pp. 539–550). Washington, DC: APA.

American Psychiatric Association. (2013). *Diagnostic and statistical manual of mental disorders* (5th ed.). Washington, DC: APA.

Bachar, E. (1998). The contributions of self psychology to the treatment of anorexia and bulimia. *American Journal of Psychotherapy, 52*(2), 147–165.

Bachar, E. (2000). The richer encounter with aggression enabled by the Kohutian approach. *Psychoanalysis and Psychotherapy, 17*(2), 23–44.

Bachar, E., Gur, E., Canetti, L., Berry, E., & Stein, D. (2010). Selflessness and perfectionism as predictors of pathological eating attitudes and disorders: A longitudinal study. *European Eating Disorders Review, 18*(6), 496–506.

Bachar, E., Kanyas, K., Latzer, Y., Bonne, O., & Lerrer, B. (2008). Depressive tendencies and lower levels of self-sacrifice in mothers, and selflessness in their anorexic daughters. *European Eating Disorders Review, 16*(3), 184–190.

Bachar, E., Latzer, Y., Canetti, L., Gur, E., Berry, E. M., & Bonne, E. (2002). Rejection of life in anorexic and bulimic patients. *International Journal of Eating Disorders, 31*, 43–48.

Bachar, E., Latzer, Y., Kreitler, S., & Berry, E. (1999). Empirical comparison of two psychological therapies: Self psychology and cognitive orientation in the treatment of anorexia and bulimia. *Journal of Psychotherapy, Practice and Research, 8*, 115–128.

Bachner-Melman, R., Zohar, A. H., Ebstein, R. P., & Bachar, E. (2007). The relationship between selflessness levels and the severity of anorexia nervosa symptomatology. *European Eating Disorders Review, 15*(3), 213–220.

Barth, D. (1991). When the patient abuses food. In H. Jackson (Ed.), *Using self psychology in psychotherapy* (pp. 223–241). London: Jason Aronson.

Bion, W. R. (1959). Attacks on linking. *International Journal of Psychoanalysis, 40*, 308–315.

Bollas, C. (1987). *The shadow of the object*. London: Free Association Books.

Bordo, S. (1993). *Unbearable weight: Feminism, Western culture, and the body*. Berkeley: University of California Press.

Boskind-Lodahl, M. (1976). Cinderella's step-sisters: A feminist perspective on anorexia nervosa and bulimia. *Signs, 2*(2), 342–356.

Brandchaft, B., & Stolorow, R. (1984). A current perspective on difficult patients. In E. Stepansky & A. Goldberg (Eds.), *Kohut's legacy* (pp. 93–115). New York: The Analytic Press.

Breuer, J., & Freud, S. (1895). Studies on hysteria. In J. Strachey (Ed. & Trans.), *The standard edition of the complete psychological works of Sigmund Freud* (Vol. II.).

Bromberg, P. (2006). *Awakening the dreamer*. Mahwah, NJ: The Analytic Press.

Bruch, H. (1970). Psychotherapy in primary anorexia nervosa. *Journal of Nervous and Mental Diseases, 150*, 51–66.

Bruch, H. (1973). *Eating disorders: Obesity, anorexia nervosa and the person within*. New York: Basic Books.

Bruch, H. (1985). Four decades of eating disorders. In D. M. Garner & P. E. Garfinkel (Eds.), *Handbook of psychotherapy for anorexia nervosa and bulimia* (pp. 7–18). New York: The Guilford Press.

Bruch, H. (1988). *Conversations with anorexics*. London: Jason Aronson.

Brunton, J. N., Lacey, J. H., & Waller, G. (2005). Narcissism and eating characteristics in young nonclinical women. *Journal of Nervous and Mental Disease, 193*, 140–143.

Chaiken, S., & Pliner, P. (1987). Women, but not men, are what they eat: The effect of meal size and gender on perceived femininity and masculinity. *Personality and Social Psychology Bulletin, 13*, 166–176.

Epstein, L. (1987). The problem of bad-analyst feeling. *Modern Psychoanalysis, 12*, 35–45.

Fingeret, M. C., Warren, C. S., Cepeda-Benito, A., & Gleaves, D. H. (2006). Eating disorder prevention research: A meta-analysis. *Eating Disorders, 14*, 191–213.

Fink, B. (2016). Compulsive eating and the death drive. In B. Fink (Ed.), *Against understanding* (pp. 58–63). London & New York: Routledge.

Franko, D. L., & Rolfe, S. (1996). Countertransference in the treatment of patients with eating disorders. *Psychiatry, 59*, 108–116.

Freud, S., Bonaparte, M., Freud, A., & Kris, E. (Eds.). (1954). *The origins of psycho-analysis: Letters to Wilhelm Fliess, drafts and notes: 1887–1902* (E. Mosbacher & J. Strachey, Trans.). New York: Basic Books.

Garner, D. M., & Garfinkel, P. E. (1985). Cognitive treatment of anorexia. In D. M. Garner & E. Garfinkel (Eds.), *Handbook of psychotherapy for anorexia nervosa and bulimia* (pp. 121–136). New York: The Guilford Press.

Geist, R. A. (1989). Self psychological reflections on the origins of eating disorders. *The Journal of the American Academy of Psychoanalysis, 17*(1), 5–28.

Gluck, M. (2000, May). *Body dissatisfaction and eating behaviors: Orthodox vs. secular Jewish women*. Paper presented at the Ninth International Conference on Eating Disorders, New York.

Goodsitt, A. (1985). Self psychology and the treatment of anorexia nervosa. In D. M. Garner & P. E. Garfinkel (Eds.), *Handbook of psychotherapy for anorexia nervosa and bulimia* (pp. 55–82). New York: The Guilford Press.

Goodsitt, A. (1997). Eating disorders: A self-psychological perspective. In D. M. Garner & P. E. Garfinkel (Eds.), *Handbook of psychotherapy for eating disorders* (2nd ed., pp. 205–228). New York: The Guilford Press.

Graves, T. A., Tabri, N., Thompson-Brenner, H., Franko, D. L., Eddy, K. T., Bourion-Bedes, S., . . . Thomas, J. J. (2017). A meta-analysis of the relation between therapeutic alliance and treatment outcome in eating disorders. *International Journal of Eating Disorders, 50*(4), 323–340.

Green, A. (2001). The dead mother. In A. Green (Ed.), *Life narcissism death narcissism* (pp. 88–101). London: Free Association Books.

Hoek, H. W. (1998, May). *Research update.* Paper presented at the Eighth International Conference on Eating Disorders, New York.

Hoek, H. W. (2006). Incidence, prevalence and mortality of anorexia nervosa and other eating disorders. *Current Opinion in Psychiatry, 19*(4), 389–394.

Hsu, G. L. K. (1990). *Eating disorders.* New York: The Guilford Press.

Kearney-Cooke, A. (1991). Men, body image and eating disorders. In A. E. Anderson (Ed.), *Males with eating disorders* (pp. 54–75). New York: Brunner/Mazel.

Klein, M. (1957). Envy and gratitude. In M. Klein (Ed.), *Envy and gratitude and other works* (pp. 176–236). London: Hogarth Press.

Kogan, C. (2011). Being a selfobject – the story of Genesis. *Sihot, 25,* 276–282.

Kohut, H. (1968). The psychoanalytic treatment of narcissistic personality disorders: Outline of a systematic approach. *Psychoanalytic Studies of the Child, 23,* 86–113.

Kohut, H. (1971). *The analysis of the self.* New York: International Universities Press.

Kohut, H. (1977a). Preface to psychodynamics of drug dependence. In J. D. Blaine & D. A. Julius (Eds.), *Psychodynamics of drug dependence* (pp. 3–10). Washington, DC: Government Printing Office.

Kohut, H. (1977b). *The restoration of the self.* New York: International Universities Press.

Kohut, H. (1979). The two analyses of Mr. Z. *International Journal of Psychoanalysis, 60,* 3–27.

Kohut, H. (1984). *How does analysis cure?* Chicago: University of Chicago Press.

Kohut, H. (1987a). Building psychic structure that regulates self-esteem. In M. Elson (Ed.), *The Kohut's seminars on self psychology and psychotherapy with adolescents and young adults* (pp. 61–76). New York: W. W. Norton & Company.

Kohut, H. (1987b). Addictive need for an admiring other in regulation of self-esteem. In M. Elson (Ed.), *The Kohut's seminars on self psychology and psychotherapy with adolescents and young adults* (pp. 113–132). New York: W. W. Norton & Company.

Kohut, H. (2011). Letters. In P. Ornstein (Ed.), *The search for the self: Selected writings of Heinz Kohut 1950-1978* (Vol. 4, pp. 669–674). London: Karnac.

Kohut, H., & Wolf, E. S. (1978). The disorders of the self and their treatment: An outline. *International Journal of Psychoanalysis*, *59*, 413–425.

Kreitler, S., Bachar, E., Canetti, L., Berry, E., & Bonne, O. (2003). The cognitive-orientation theory of anorexia nervosa. *Journal of Clinical Psychology*, *59*, 651–671.

Kulka, R. (2005). Between tragedy and compassion: Introduction essay. In H. Kohut (Ed.), *How does analysis cure* (E. Eidan, Trans.) (pp. 13–52). Tel Aviv: Am Oved.

Leung, F., David, C., & Cheung, P. (1998, May). *The ideal woman's body-figure among Chinese in Hong Kong*. Paper presented at the Eighth International Conference on Eating Disorders, New York.

Levin, J. (1991). When the patient abuses alcohol. In H. Jackson (Ed.), *Using self psychology in psychotherapy* (pp. 203–221). London: Jason Aronson.

Levin, M. P. (1994). Beauty myth and the beast: What men can do and be to help prevent eating disorders. *Eating Disorders: The Journal of Treatment and Prevention*, *2*(2), 101–113.

Levin, M. P., & Smolak, L. (1992). Toward a model of the development of psychopathology of eating disorders: The example of early adolescence. In J. H. Crowther, D. L. Tennenbaum, S. E. Hobfoll, & M. A. P. Stephens (Eds.), *The etiology of bulimia nervosa: The individual and familial context* (pp. 59–80). Washington, DC: Taylor & Francis.

Macsween, M. (1993). *Anorexic bodies: A feminist and sociological perspective on anorexia nervosa*. New York: Routledge.

Mahler, M. (1968). *On human symbiosis and the vicissitudes of individuation*. New York: International Universities Press.

Mahler, M. (1975). *The psychological birth of the human infant*. New York: Basic Books.

Masserman, J. H. (1941). Psychodynamics in anorexia nervosa and neurotic vomiting. *Psychoanalytic Quarterly*, *10*, 211–242.

Masterson, J. F. (1976). *Psychotherapy of the borderline adult: A developmental approach*. New York: Brunner/Mazel.

Masterson, J. F. (1995). Paradise lost – bulimia, a closet narcissistic personality disorder: A developmental, self, and object relations approach. In R. C. Marohn & S. C. Feinstein (Eds.), *Adolescent psychiatry* (pp. 253–266). New York: The Analytic Press.

Medina-Pradas, C., Navarro, J. B., López, S. R., Grau, A., & Obiols, J. E. (2011). Dyadic view of expressed emotion, stress, and eating disorder psychopathology. *Appetite*, *57*(3), 743–748.

Minuchin, S., Rosman, B. L., & Baker, L. (1978). *Psychosomatic families*. Cambridge, MA: Harvard University Press.

Modell, A. (1971). The origins of certain forms of pre-oedipal guilt and the implications for a psychoanalytical theory of affects. *International Journal of Psychoanalysis*, *52*, 337–345.

Morton, R. (1694). *Physiology of consumption* (Vol. 2, pp. 5–6). London: Smith & Walford.

Moulton, R. (1942). A psychosomatic study of anorexia nervosa including the use of vaginal smears. *Psychosomatic Medicine, 4,* 62–74.

Neumark, D. S., Butler, R., & Palti, H. (1995). Eating disturbances among adolescent girls: Evaluation of a school-based primary prevention program. *Journal of Nutrition Education, 27,* 24–31.

Newman, K. (1980). Defense analysis and self psychology. In A. Goldberg (Ed.), *Advances in self psychology* (pp. 263–278). New York: International Universities Press.

Orbach, S. (1986). *Hunger strike: The anorectic's struggle as a metaphor for our age.* New York: W. W. Norton & Company.

Ornstein, A. (1990). Selfobject transferences and the process of working through. *Progress in Self Psychology, 6,* 41–58.

Petrucelli, J. (2015). 'My body is a cage': Interfacing interpersonal neurobiology, attachment, affect regulation, self-regulation, and the regulation of relatedness in treatment with patients with eating disorders. In J. Petrucelli (Ed.), *Body states: Interpersonal and relational perspectives on the treatment of eating disorders* (pp. 35–56). New York: Routledge.

Pinus, U., Canetti, L., Bonne, O., & Bachar, E. (2019). Selflessness as a predictor of remission from an eating disorder: 1–4 Year outcomes from an adolescent day-care unit. *Eating and Weight Disorders–Studies on Anorexia, Bulimia and Obesity, 24*(4), 777–786.

Sands, S. (1989). Eating disorders and female development: A self-psychological perspective. *Progress in Self Psychology, 5,* 75–103.

Sands, S. (1991). Bulimia, dissociation and empathy: A self-psychological view. In C. Johnson (Ed.), *Psychodynamic treatment of anorexia nervosa and bulimia nervosa* (pp. 34–50). New York: The Guilford Press.

Sands, S. (2003). The subjugation of the body in eating disorders: A particularly female solution. *Psychoanalytic Psychology, 20*(1), 103–116.

Schwaber, E. (1984). A mode of analytic listening. In J. Lichtenberg, M. Bronstein, & D. Silver (Eds.), *Empathy* (pp. 143–172). New York: The Analytic Press.

Selvini-Palazzoli, M. (1985). *Self-starvation: From individual to family therapy in the treatment of anorexia nervosa.* London: Jason Aronson.

Silverstein, B., & Perlick, D. (1995). *The cost of competence: Why inequality causes depression, eating disorders and illness in women.* New York: Oxford University Press.

Slochower, J. (1991). Variations in the analytic holding environment. *International Journal of Psychoanalysis, 72,* 709–714.

Sours, J. A. (1980). *Starving to death in a sea of objects: The anorexia nervosa syndrome.* London: Jason Aronson.

Strober, M. (1998, May). *Long-term outcome in anorexia nervosa: Survival analysis of recovery, relapse and outcome predictors in a 10–15 years prospective.* Paper presented at the Eighth International Conference on Eating Disorders, New York.

Swift, W. J. (1991). Bruch revisited: The role of interpretation of transference and resistance in the psychotherapy of eating disorders. In C. Johnson (Ed.), *Psychodynamic treatment of anorexia nervosa and bulimia nervosa* (pp. 51–66). New York: The Guilford Press.

Tchanturia, K., & Katzman, M. (2000, May). *A post-communist country with a capitalist problem? Experiences of eating disorders in Georgia from Soviet Union.* Paper presented at the Ninth International Conference on Eating Disorders, New York.

Tolpin, M. (1980). Discussion of "Self psychology and the concept of psychopathology: A case presentation" by Evelyne A. Schwaber. In A. Goldberg (Ed.), *Advances in self psychology* (pp. 243–251). New York: International Universities Press.

Thompson-Brenner, H., Satir, D. A., Franko, D. L., & Herzog, D. B. (2012). Clinician reactions to patients with eating disorders: A review of the literature. *Psychiatric Services, 63*(1), 73–78.

Ulman, R. B., & Paul, H. (1989). A self-psychological theory and approach to treating substance abuse disorders: The intersubjective absorption hypothesis. *Progress in Self Psychology, 5,* 121–141.

Verbin, A. (2016). *Notes from the looking glass land: Body and subjectivity in memoirs of anorectic women.* (Thesis for the degree of Doctor of Philosophy), Hebrew University, Jerusalem, Israel.

Waller, J. V., Kaufman, M. R., & Deutsch, F. (1940). Anorexia nervosa: A psychodynamic entity. *Psychosomatic Medicine, 2,* 3–16.

Wechselblatt, T., Gurnick, G., & Simon, R. (2000). Autonomy and relatedness in the development of anorexia nervosa: A clinical case series using grounded theory. *Bulletin of the Menninger Clinic, 64*(1), 91–123.

Williams, G. (1997). *Internal landscapes and foreign bodies, eating disorders and other pathologies.* London: Duckworth.

Winnicott, D. W. (1965a). The development of the capacity for concern. In D. W. Winnicott (Ed.), *The maturation processes and the facilitating environment* (pp. 73–82). London: Hogarth Press.

Winnicott, D. W. (1965b). From dependence towards independence in the development of the individual. In D. W. Winnicott (Ed.), *The maturation processes and the facilitating environment* (pp. 83–92). London: Hogarth Press.

Wolf, E. (1988). *Treating the self: Elements of clinical self psychology.* New York: The Guilford Press.

Wolf, E. (1995). *Concepts in self psychology: Theory and clinical practice* (pp. 13–27). Jerusalem: Summit Institute.

Zipfel, S., Wild, B., Gross, G., Friederich, H. C., Teufel, M., Scehllberg, D., . . . Herzog, W. (2014). Focal psychodynamic therapy, cognitive behavior therapy, and optimized treatment as usual in outpatients with anorexia nervosa (ANTOP study): Randomised controlled trial. *Lancet, 383,* 127–137.

Index

For Product Safety Concerns and Information please contact our EU
representative GPSR@taylorandfrancis.com Taylor & Francis Verlag GmbH,
Kaufingerstraße 24, 80331 München, Germany

Printed and bound by CPI Group (UK) Ltd, Croydon, CR0 4YY
08/06/2025
01897007-0004